ACKNOWLEDGEMENTS BY PARTICIPATING CAESAREAN MOTHERS

. . . .

"Thank you for this book – a great idea. Thank you for your work and initiative. You helped me accept my ‚Caesarean fate' in its entirety."

47 YEARS, 1 CAESAREAN

. . . .

"A book by women – for women!"

35 YEARS, 1 CAESAREAN

. . . .

"It is always good to chat to other Caesarean mothers and, despite all the different experiences, to come to the conclusion that this was the best way to deliver a healthy child! Good luck with your book!"

36 YEARS, 2 CAESAREANS

. . . .

"It feels so good to be able to share experiences with like-minded people."

50 YEARS, 2 CAESAREANS

. . . .

"Through this project I have been able to remember a lot of things that I experienced 40 years ago. An interesting project!"

65 YEARS, 2 CAESAREANS

. . . .

"Good luck with the book! I think this is exactly what expectant mummies need."

28 YEARS, 2 CHILDREN, 1 CAESAREAN

. . . .

"The scar on the outside is not the same as the inner scar – Thanks for the experience."

29 YEARS, 3 CAESAREANS

Caroline Oblasser

Photographs by Gudrun Wesp

C-Section Moms

Caesarean mothers in words and photographs

Photo book, guide and
a treasure trove of experiences
for pregnant women, mothers
and obstetricians

Introduction by Marsden Wagner MD, MS
Critical Comment by Gretchen Humphries, MS DVM

• •

Translated by Claudia Pichler

• •

We want to thank our medical consultants who supported the translation:
Anna Rockel-Loenhoff, Midwife/Physician, Midwife Trainer, European Institute of Midwifery
Elizabeth Hormann, Ed.M., IBCLC
Malcolm Griffiths MD, FRCOG • Sadek Pharaon MD, FRCOG
Dr Fiona Schneider, FRCOG • Nicole Zenner, MRCOG, IBCLC
Florian Drews MD, Specialty Registrar in Obstetrics and Gynaecology

edition
riedenburg

Bibliografische Information der Deutschen Nationalbibliothek
Die Deutsche Nationalbibliothek verzeichnet diese Publikation in der Deutschen Nationalbibliografie;
detaillierte bibliografische Daten sind im Internet über
http://dnb.d-nb.de abrufbar.

Second Edition – 2014
© 2009–2014   edition riedenburg • Salzburg • Austria
Address   edition riedenburg • Anton-Hochmuth-Strasse 8 • 5020 Salzburg • Austria
E-Mail   verlag@editionriedenburg.at
Website   www.editionriedenburg.at

Credits
Photographs   Gudrun Wesp, www.goWesp.at
Cover Illustration   © Stauke – Fotolia.com

Layout   edition riedenburg
Publisher   edition riedenburg, editionriedenburg.at

ISBN 978-3-902943-52-1

Contents

Introduction by Marsden Wagner MD, MS

At Last! After years of obstetricians telling women the wonders of Caesarean sections – "bikini cut", "gentle" Caesareans, etc., etc. – someone has finally asked the women who have had all these Caesareans whether or not they are, in fact, so wonderful. And surprise – they are anything but wonderful. This book documents in personal statements and photos the reality of Caesareans as experienced by the women.

42 % of women describe their Caesareans as "traumatic" and one-third had health problems after their Caesareans. They did not experience their Caesareans as either pain free nor quick. The photos expose the truth about the Caesarean scar – many of the scars are deforming and many women have difficulty adjusting their self concept to incorporate the new scar.

Nearly all of the women in the book agree the media is complicit with the obstetricians in trivializing Caesareans and not telling the women the truth – this procedure is major abdominal surgery with serious risks both for the woman and her baby. In 1985 the World Health Organization (WHO), after reviewing the world's scientific literature, recommended 15 % of all births as Caesareans as the upper limit of safety and in 2007 WHO, after reviewing all national Caesarean rates, reaffirmed 15% as the upper limit beyond which the maternal mortality rises.

Doing unnecessary Caesareans increases the number of women dying as research has proven that "scheduled" Caesareans (no medical emergency) have over double the risk of maternal death than vaginal birth. So as the rate of Caesareans in many developed countries increases to 20 % and then 25 % and now over 30 % in some countries, hundreds and hundreds of women are dying unnecessarily. Women are not told this truth either by their care givers nor the media, they are told the lie that Caesarean birth is just as safe as vaginal birth. Women seem to know this intuitively as nearly all of the women surveyed in this book felt that while Caesareans were necessary in the case of a medical emergency, vaginal birth was otherwise to be preferred.

Women must also be told the truth about the increased risks for their baby if the birth is Caesarean rather than vaginal. In 9 % of the cases in this book, when the scalpel cut through the uterine wall to get the baby out, it also cut into the baby. Considerable research has shown that the risk that the baby will die after a Caesarean is significantly higher than after a vaginal birth due to respiratory distress and/or prematurity. But the women were not told these important truths about the risks of Caesarean to their baby.

This book also shows that women who have had a cesarean understand the truth that the cause of the rising rate of Caesarean births is not the wishes of women, but the wishes of doctors. For doctors to say that more and more women choose Caesarean is yet another lie to cover up their own needs for the convenience of scheduling Caesareans, making more money and avoiding litigation. You can't fool women all the time.

The births described by the women in this book reveals some of the bad maternity care practices they experienced. Many of these women had their labor induced for no scientifically valid reason and it is this very induction which has been proven to be one of the causes of excessive Caesarean sections. In addition, the scientific evidence is clear – with a Caesarean section in which the woman has an epidural and is awake and alert, the baby should be given to the woman immediately at birth for skin-to-skin contact and bonding before the baby is examined and clothed. This occurred in almost none of the cases in this book.

The book finishes with an excellent set of recommendations for teaching pregnant women how to cope with the possibility that they will be told at the time of giving birth that they need a Caesarean.

And including the photos of a "gentle" birth in the book is excellent as it makes it clear to the reader that a Caesarean is indeed major abdominal surgery and can never be labeled "gentle". The more the women in this book were educated during pregnancy about the reality of Caesarean, the fewer experienced their subsequent Caesarean as traumatic. Women need the bare truth, not sweet talk.

This book should be read by all pregnant women as it speaks the bare truth.

Marsden Wagner, MD, MS, is a perinatologist, neonatalogist and perinatal epidemiologist from California who is an outspoken supporter of midwifery. He was responsible for maternal and child health in the European Regional Office of WHO for 14 years. Marsden travels all over the world to talk about appropriate uses of technology in birth and utilizing midwives for the best outcome. His books "Born in the USA: How a broken maternity care system must be fixed to put women and children first." and "Creating Your Birth Plan: The definitive Guide to a Safe and Empowering Birth" are a must for anyone involved in birth.

Critical Comment by Gretchen Humphries, MS DVM

Everyone knows that Caesareans save lives. But what many people don't understand or accept is that they can ruin lives too.

A Caesarean is not "just another way to have a baby" nor is it the "painless" option we so often hear about in the popular media and mainstream online message boards. In 2006, in the United States, at least 31.1 % of all babies were delivered via major abdominal surgery (the accuracy of this number is suspect, since many states do not report Caesareans that were performed because of a breech presentation or multiples, or any other "high risk" complication to the pregnancy – the true Caesarean rate in the U.S may be significantly higher). Many of these new mothers were left with questions about how they ended up with a Caesarean and feelings of confusion, isolation and regret.

It is strangely acceptable to share "war stories" about the horrors of birth (particularly vaginal birth) but any ambivalence about the necessity of what ultimately occurred during the birth is met with a vehement "all that matters is a healthy baby" and criticism that any woman could be so selfish as to question the necessity of her Caesarean. The belief that doctor knows best and only has the best interest of the mother and baby in mind is a hard belief to let go.

While the catch phrase "too posh to push" may have originated in the United Kingdom, the notion that women are somehow forcing their obstetricians to give them unnecessary and potentially dangerous Caesareans without any medical reason has been gleefully promulgated throughout American popular culture, with not a shred of evidence to support its truth. Like the women in this book, women in the U.S. are not requesting elective surgery for no reason. Nor are more women needing Caesareans because they are old or fat or carrying babies conceived through fertility treatments.

As the women in this book know, the reasons for the increase in Caesareans are more about how healthy women are being misled, about how the medical profession stands to benefit both financially and legally and about how the whole reality of what childbirth is has been warped into something that more resembles cancer or infection than a natural physiological function. Unfortunately, it is those with the least amount of power in our culture that suffer from this epidemic of Caesareans – the women and their children. As is often the case, it is easier to blame the victim than take responsibility for the harm being done.

Fortunately, the same global connectedness that makes the apparently shallow choice of a pop-star in the U.K. to schedule non-medically indicated surgery an example of modern motherhood also allows a different view to emerge. Women are discovering that they aren't alone in their disquiet over their Caesareans.

The strength and sorrow of "C-Section Moms" is that it IS so many women. The stories you will read here are the stories of millions of women. They are stories I hear every day in my work with the International Caesarean Awareness Network (ICAN). Not every woman is upset about her Caesarean and not every Caesarean is suspect. But even with a necessary, life-saving cesarean, the feelings that can follow are complex and deserve both respect and a wider understanding.

> "We need to tell true stories about caesareans, so that those who come after us aren't caught off guard the way so many of us were."

The one characteristic I see in all the women I work with is that they are willing to do whatever they believe is best for their babies and their families. That willingness to sacrifice for a child is being taken advantage of by a medical profession too absorbed with its own concerns to remember the oath "First do no harm"; women and babies are being harmed, every single day.

My hope for "C-Section Moms" is that it will be widely read, particularly by women who have not yet had to negotiate the complexities of modern maternity care. Most of the women I know who had a Caesarean never expected one and the truth is, right now any pregnant woman has a very real chance of having a Caesarean, no matter what her pregnancy is like, no matter what her previous births may have been like.

We need to tell true stories about Caesareans, so that those who come after us aren't caught off guard the way so many of us were. If the medical professionals, hospital administrators and insurance adjustors responsible for the increasing number of Caesareans also read this book and get a glimpse of the ongoing pain they are at least partly responsible for, even better. If a woman who thought she was "the only one who felt that way about my Caesarean" reads this and finds her voice to speak out and make a difference then we will all benefit.

After a decade working with ICAN to prevent unnecessary Caesareans, promote vaginal birth after Caesarean (VBAC) and provide support for Caesarean recovery, I believe it will only change when women say "enough is enough and we won't lay down for this anymore".

Gretchen Humphries, MS DVM is the Advocacy Director for the International Caesarean Awareness Network (ICAN) and has been working with women who've had Caesareans for 10 years, providing support for women recovering from a Caesarean, planning a vaginal birth after Caesarean (VBAC) or trying to avoid an unnecessary Caesarean. She is the mother of 4 children and practices Veterinary Medicine at an Emergency and Critical Care Hospital in Michigan, United States. She is the author of numerous essays, many of which can be found at www.birthtruth.org. She is an invited speaker on various topics relating to Caesareans and VBAC and represents ICAN and its constituents with various midwifery and other birth-related advocacy groups. She is a contributing author to "Cesarean Voices", a collection of first-person accounts about the Caesarean experience, a book that should be read by anyone touched by a Caesarean, either personally or professionally. Her latest project quantified the increase in the number of hospitals in the United States that formally "ban" VBAC from their facility, leaving women with no option other than a repeat Caesarean.

Website of ICAN: www.ican-online.org

Understand all the Choices you have!

Debra Pascali-Bonaro („Orgasmic Birth") on Caesarean section and Normal Birth

A must see and read book for all expectant women, their partners, childbirth educators, doulas, nurses, and all who care for childbearing women! The powerful images of the scars of Caesarean birth on women's bodies in combination with women's words uncover the marks that are left on mother's physical and emotional well-being for years to come. A deeply moving and informative portrayal of a far too common procedure in childbirth today.

C-Section Moms provides readers with a great deal of information, which makes them consider where, with whom and how we birth our babies and the effect our choices have. I hope that every woman reads this book and then visits the Website **www.thebirthsurvey.com** to learn what their provider and facility's rates of interventions are.

Most people are informed consumers and would never buy a cell phone, computer or car without knowing detailed information about all their options. It is time women begin to ask questions and understand what model of care they are being offered, and the outcomes and options available to them in labor and birth. For example, if a woman's provider/facility has a 40 % rate of Caesarean birth, that also becomes her rate, while there may be other providers who work with low risk women in the region and have a rate of fewer than 10 % or even 5 %. You and your baby deserve to have a safe, satisfying and pleasurable birth.

While Caesarean surgery can be life saving when needed, we must question the overuse of technology and surgery and the effect it is having on mothers and babies in relation to both their short and long term health and well being. An aspect of the book that I find very important is that the reader is able to learn the elements of having a positive Caesarean birth that include informed decision making, respect, nurturing, support, and when a Caesarean section is needed how her providers can help a woman to have a "gentle Caesarean section" that preserves and protects her memory of birth and maintains birth as a positive experience. A woman's memory of her birth will last a life time. Women deserve to have a positive experience under any situation.

Women should also consider the many underused and cost effective options that can reduce the incidence of Caesarean section. Lamaze International has created **The Six Care Practices that Support Normal Birth** (**www.lamaze.org**).

They include

- labor beginning on it's own,
- freedom of movement throughout labor,
- continuous support,
- no routine interventions,
- spontaneous pushing in upright or gravity-neutral positions, and
- no separation of mother and baby after birth with unlimited opportunities for breastfeeding.

Simple techniques such as the use of water, touch, massage, dimming lights and creating a safe, sensuous atmosphere can help to make labor easier, thus reducing the need for interventions that often lead to Caesarean surgery.

The ability to have continuous support during labor and birth, including doulas, has many well-documented benefits and can reduce the rate of Caesarean birth.

"If you don't know your options you don't have any."

DONA International describes a birth doula as "a person trained and experienced in childbirth who provides continuous physical, emotional and informational support to the mother and her partner before, during and just after childbirth."

Numerous clinical studies have found that a doula's presence at birth:

- tends to result in shorter labors with fewer complications,
- reduces negative feelings about one's childbirth experience,
- reduces the need for pitocin (a labor-inducing drug), forceps or vacuum extraction,
- reduces the requests for pain medication and epidurals, as well as the incidence of Caesareans

Childbirth Connection's new report **New Mothers Speak Out** shows us disturbing data about new mothers in the United States. Validated mental health screening tools found that around the time of the follow-up survey most mothers (63 %) were likely to be experiencing some degree of depressive symptoms, and 18 % appeared to be experiencing some symptoms of post-traumatic stress with reference to their childbirth experience.

A time in a woman's life that has the potential to be ecstatic or as I have learned even "Orgasmic", is turning traumatic for far too many new mothers and often these are women who experience technology driven births, including assisted births and Caesarean sections.

Visit **www.childbirthconnection.org/listeningtomothers** to read all three Listening to Mothers reports.

As a doula, childbirth educator and Director of the documentary **Orgasmic Birth**, I have often said, "if you don't know your options you don't have any."

It is time women understand all the choices that are being offered to them, the benefits and harms of each and how their decicision will effect them for the rest of their lives.

C-Section Moms provides an important contribution to creating the awareness of the benefits and harms that Caesarean surgery poses to women and their babies and helping women to make informed decisions about their care.

Debra Pascali-Bonaro LCCE, CD (DONA), is an internationally respected childbirth expert, a 26-year speaker in childbirth education, and a Lamaze-certified veteran in maternity care with a passion for birth. She is the mother of three sons and two stepchildren. Debra is Co-Chair of the International MotherBaby Childbirth Initiative, which works in collaboration with global leaders and groups to reduce maternal and infant mortality and improve care for mothers, babies, and families. She serves on the Board of Directors for Childbirth Connection and is a DONA-approved doula trainer. She coauthored *Nurturing Beginnings: Mother Love's Guide to Postpartum Home Care for Doulas and Outreach Workers* and received Lamaze International's Elizabeth Bing Award in 2002. Debra began videotaping births worldwide in 2002 as she traveled to New Zealand, Mexico, the U.K., and South America, and throughout the United States in her birth outreach work. Orgasmic Birth is her first film.

Websites:
www.motherlovedoulas.com; International MotherBaby Childbirth Initiative: www.imbci.org; Orgasmic Birth: www.orgasmicbirth.com

The author's preface

162 Caesarean mothers, 60 of them featured in words and photographs, make this photo book a special and very personal reference guide. It cannot and will not give a definitive presentation of the phenomenon "Caesarean section", but rather a presentation as critical and as comprehensive as possible.

All women remain anonymous within the book. There are no faces, exact dates of birth or names. Where necessary, I neutralised data that were too personal or would allow specific conclusions to be drawn.

Nowadays, in these rapidly changing times influenced by outside factors like the media, I find it necessary and meaningful to make available to all the valuable and complex Caesarean experiences of those personally concerned and involved.

This is available to all who

- want to deal with this way of delivery consciously

- have experienced one or more Caesarean sections themselves and are curious about other people's experiences

- want to understand the effect of the Caesarean on mother and child.

The Caesarean photo book would not be a "photo book" if it did not show

- what the Caesarean scar, which is, to some extent, trivialised as a "bikini scar", looks like after one or more Caesarean surgeries.

I want the research to give the Caesarean section a manifold "face" and help it out of its sometimes simplified predicament shaped by modernism.

May the Caesarean again become what it is supposed to be according to almost all the participants of this photo book: A surgical measure, which saves the life of a mother and the life of her child in an emergency.

Salzburg, April 2014
Caroline Oblasser

The Caesarean section:

Fantastic or traumatic?

If a Caesarean section suddenly becomes necessary during delivery many women feel taken by surprise because this way of delivery is mostly not a central topic in antenatal classes; furthermore, the attending obstetrician has usually not dealt with it extensively during checkups. Everything had indicated a quick and trouble-free birth following a normal pregnancy...

If the Caesarean has to be performed under general anaesthetic due to a lack of time, many mothers only catch a glimpse of their baby hours later. The first breastfeeding during the hormonal high after birth remains an unfulfilled dream, one's own child seems oddly strange – as he or she is handed over fully dressed and not placed naked on the mother's tummy in the delivery room.

In addition to the postoperative pain, mothers who have gone through an emergency Caesarean often have the feeling of having "failed" and not having done everything for the child, even though intensive labour as well as a strong belief in being able to manage the natural way, often precede the surgical outcome of the birth.

Other pregnant women engage in a more or less planned Caesarean section for reasons which up-to-date medical research or medical skills identify, be it a breech presentation (the legs or the buttocks present before the head), circumstances which (seem to) make a spontaneous birth impossible or the presence of a multiple pregnancy.

In all these cases, the mother-to-be is usually at least basically informed about the upcoming event and often makes use of the opportunity to "talk" to the unborn baby about the Caesarean section and to actively prepare herself for it together with the child.

The experiences of our participants in this project show that the ability to keep a positive view of the birth in mind involves being well prepared for a possible Caesarean section. Women who had the chance to deal with the "diagnosis Caesarean" for long enough prior to the abdominal delivery mostly cope with it better, in the long term, than those who change from having a healthy pregnancy into being a patient within a short time.

The elective Caesarean section and Caesareans not medically indicated

Frequently the mass media and magazines suggest that "Caesarean on demand" is the modern way of delivery for celebrities. But of course it is not only some celebrities who decide on an elective Caesarean from the beginning, "normal" women do so too.

Why is this the case? Reasons may, for example, be previous traumatic vaginal deliveries or expected complications during birth.

Inadequate education regarding the topic of Caesarean sections to date definitely plays a role; the fact that not one of our 162 Caesarean mothers had an elective Caesarean section twice in her life says a lot.

Furthermore, none of the participating mothers named convenience or better scheduling as the reason for requesting a Caesarean. The survey of experts, conducted in writing and carried out with 156 midwives, obstetricians, physicians and therapists, indicated that many obstetricians name exactly those factors mentioned above on the part of the mothers as the driving force behind the rapid increase in the rate of Caesarean sections.

To be exact almost all of the midwives interviewed, namely 96 % (!) are of the opinion that many Caesareans are performed without medical indication today. They explain the "boom" in Caesareans as follows (decreasing occurrence):

1. **Fear of birth**
   Mother: Afraid of pain, fear passed on by the obstetrician
   Obstetrician: Forensic pressure, fear of legal consequences

2. **Desire for a Caesarean section**
   Mother: Foreseeable birth, desire enforced by pressure by the media and social "trend" ("celebrities")
   Obstetrician/hospital: Timesaving, forensic exoneration, safety thinking, financial aspect

3. **Insufficient education and lack of experience**
   Obstetrician: The natural procedure of birth is thought of as being a pathological process due to lack of experience, increasing inability to conduct complicated births (e.g. breech presentation)

4. **Impatience**
   Mother: Lacking frustration tolerance, lacking stamina
   Obstetrician: Unnecessary/premature induced birth

5. **Convenience**
   Mother: Handing over the responsibility for the birth
   Obstetrician: Better scheduling of a Caesarean surgery

6. **Insufficient education in the run-up**
   Mother: Erroneous belief that the Caesarean section is the painless alternative
   Obstetrician: No mention of complications that can occur / lack of knowledge regarding possible implications

Who is right and what are the real reasons behind the obvious "trend" leading to an increase in Caesarean sections?

In trying to answer this question one has to consider that both parties – the pregnant woman and if applicable her partner as well as the obstetrician in charge – are obviously interested in experiencing or conducting the birth as quickly and as painlessly as possible and above all without endangering mother or child.

Due to the fact that lawsuits against obstetricians – who did not perform a possible Caesarean or did not perform it in time when complications occurred during birth – have increased recently, the shared wish of the pregnant woman and the medical attendant often ends in criticism and verbal attacks.

So can you accuse the obstetrician if he or she, possibly out of fear of the expected forensic complications of the delivery (and then possible legal action), recommends a Caesarean – even if there is no urgent medical indication?

And what about the cases in which the obstetrician is accused of lacking commitment and motivation e.g. during delays while giving birth, maybe even in the middle of the night? Does possible financial enrichment by doing a quick and easy Caesarean section play a role amongst obstetricians?

And seen from the obstetrician's point of view: What should be done if the pregnant woman, influenced by sugarcoated reports (of celebrities), imagines the birth to be "a walk in the park" and is not prepared for the fact that she has to cope with her body's natural power?

If contractions suddenly throw her off her guard – or long before the contractions set in, the fear of having sole responsibility for the birth? If the Caesarean section presents the more acceptable alternative for the woman? If she does not want to know about risks or possible long-term effects because she has already totally identified with this way of delivery, persists in her viewpoint and cannot be swayed? Below we want to summarise some of the results of the survey carried out on 162 Caesarean mothers.

Fear of the Caesarean section and lack of information in the run-up (4.25, 4.26, 6.1)

About 40 % of the mothers interviewed said they were afraid of a possible 1st Caesarean. About 37 % were afraid of the 2nd and about 24 % of the 3rd Caesarean. Only 27 % of the women had dealt with the abdominal delivery intensively prior to the birth. In other words: only one in four women knew roughly what to expect **before** her Caesarean surgery!

Complications after the Caesarean section (4.16)/ Breastfeeding after the Caesarean (4.17, 4.18, 4.19)

Approximately one in five women (19 %) mentioned that complications occurred during the 1st, 2nd or 3rd Caesarean section. These ranged from problems with the anaesthetic, bleeding and loss of a large amount of blood to troubles with the wound/suture and problems of the child.

The majority of the mothers (67 %) breastfed for a couple of months after the 1st Caesarean. 8 % stated that they had breastfed for more than 1 year and only 2 % of the mothers breastfed for more than 2 years. One in ten mothers did not breastfeed at all after the 1st Caesarean section.

Most of the mothers (98 %) wanted to breastfeed after the 1st Caesarean and about 73 % after the 2nd or 3rd Caesarean. After the 1st Caesarean more than one third of the women who wanted to breastfeed had problems, whereas, none of the women specified having troubles breastfeeding after the 2nd or 3rd Caesarean.

Among other things, the mothers reported lack of support when breastfeeding (bad care in hospital), sensitive nipples or inflammation, lacking milk, late first contact with the child and infant problems which led to troubles in breastfeeding.

Injuries of the child during/due to the Caesarean section (4.32)

The mother is bound to be injured during the Caesarean section because her child is delivered through the deep abdominal incision (see photo report of a "gentle" section using the Misgav Ladach method beginning on page 157). But is there also a risk for the child with a Caesarean, for example being directly affected by a cut? Absolutely yes, because 9 % of the mothers report an injury to their child (mostly cuts, scratches or marks) related to the surgery.

Possible and actual problems of a child after a Caesarean section (4.33, 4.34, 6.6)

About 40 % of the Caesarean mothers interviewed think that a Caesarean birth may possibly have negative effects on the child:

"There is a reason for natural births – of sensory importance. I think that natural births lead to the first intensive confrontation with life. Increasingly I get the feeling that with my Caesarean births I missed out on a natural end to my pregnancy – something that is indicated by mother and child, not by physicians." [T142]

"[The child] cannot get ready (before term), it gets cold – loud – bright – uncomfortable way too fast." [T129]

"Especially when the Caesarean is performed without contractions beforehand. Then the child is totally unprepared and is yanked out of the stomach. It has to be a shock!" [T055]

Research on the effects of the Caesarean birth is unavoidably still in the early stages because the generation born before us still delivered the normal way. Therefore, possible connections between a section and subsequent health problems of mother and child will only be identified in a few years or decades – and maybe by then the "trend" of Caesarean section will have moved in the opposite i.e. decreasing direction.

Once many children were not breastfed because it was assumed that breast milk was contaminated. Today many children are delivered by Caesarean section because it is reputed to be the safest way of delivery.

The Caesarean scar (5.1, 5.3)

While the word "Caesarean" resounds throughout the land, the Caesarean scar which comes with it has rarely been talked about – till now.

This 7-year-old girl's mother participated in our questionnaire:

The cut on the left cheek is approx. 2–3 mm broad and approx. 3.5 cm long
(see also [T113] on page 118).

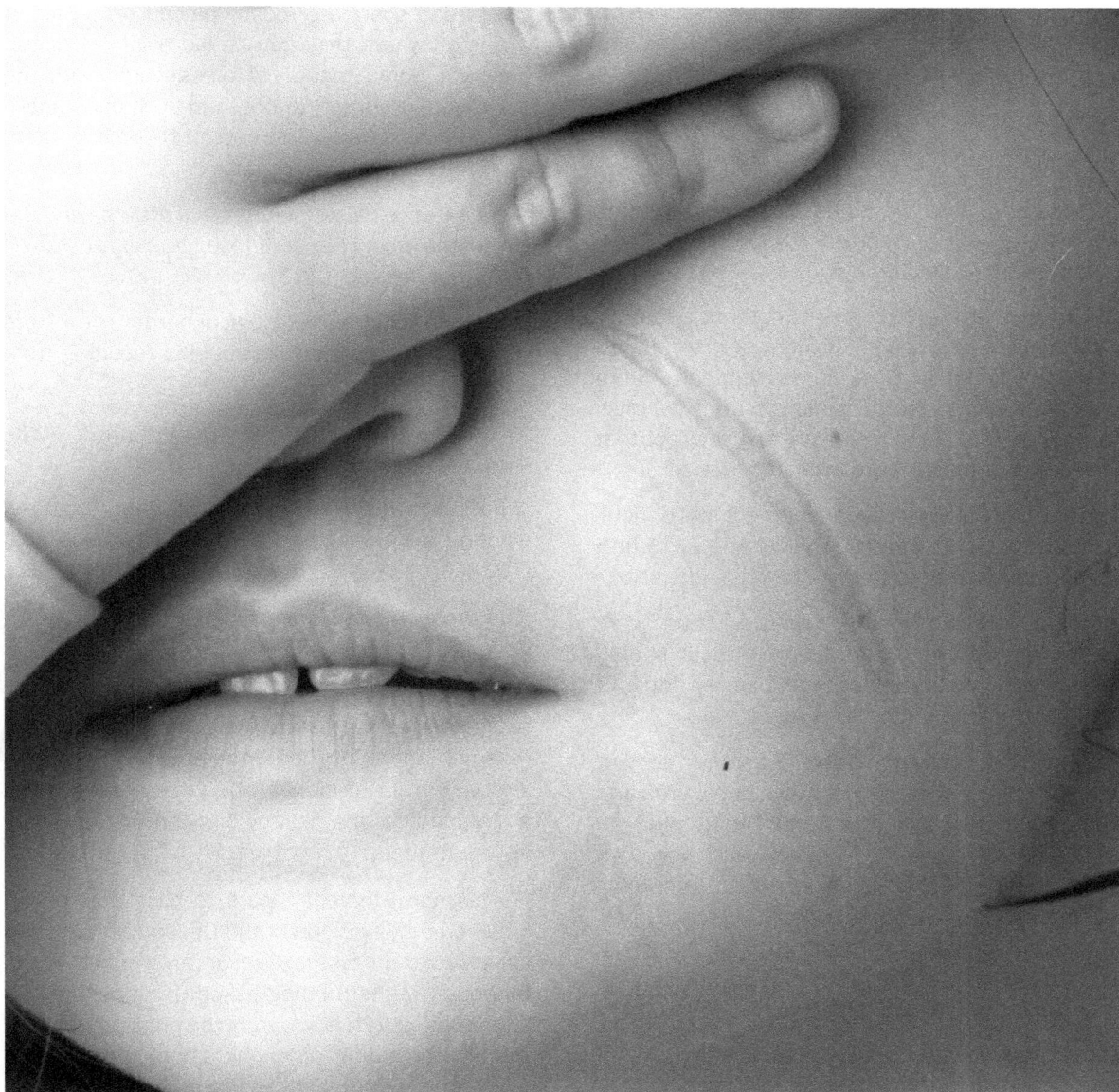

The Caesarean section: Fantastic or traumatic?

In reality it is actually the Caesarean scar which day after day reminds every Caesarean mother of her child's birth. This scar is on an intimate part of the body and is approximately 15 cm long, which is the length of a ball point pen or the distance between the thumb and the index finger.

Approximately one in five women (19 %) said that their Caesarean scar did not heal without problems. Complications ranged from scar adhesion to sensitivity in the area surrounding the scar and an unaesthetic appearance of the scar.

More than half of the mothers (59 %) said that they can feel their Caesarean scar. They mostly talked about a sharp pain, itching or sensitivity to changes in weather. Since the surgery wearing lacey underwear or tight pants is no longer possible for some Caesarean mothers.

One in four of the Caesarean mothers finds her Caesarean scar "ugly". Furthermore, we heard diverse comparisons and descriptions: From "shaped like a plate" to "smiling", from "whimsical" to "grim". The "bikini scar" and the fact that the scar is "bulging" were often mentioned.

One in four of the Caesarean mothers has difficulty in accepting her Caesarean scar and every fifth woman said she does not like touching the scar.

If the Caesarean section is propagated as a "gentle" delivery option, the Caesarean scar should definitely be discussed as well, like the topic of the pelvic floor, prior to the surgery.

When preparing for an elective Caesarean section we recommend shaving one's own pubic area and placing a 15 cm long and 5 mm broad band-aid parallel to the hair line. This band-aid is then worn non-stop for a couple of weeks – also when having intercourse – and if necessary renewed. Afterwards you decide for yourself whether you would like to keep your "scar" for the rest of your life – or, as you have the choice, rather not.

Should you decide on the latter, simply take off the band-aid and throw it in the rubbish bin.

Please don't forget that, when simulating with the band-aid, this is only attached to the surface of the skin. In reality it is not just your skin that is "stitched together" after a Caesarean but also the layers below (see sketch on page 158). To get an impression of the desired surgery read from page 159 of this book and imagine being the patient on the operating table.

Caesarean scars are mostly placed on a part of the body where they can cause a lot of "disturbances": Some meridians are severed with the conventional surgery (more than 90 % of our interviewees had a transverse cut) and even if mothers have these scars treated later on, ...

"I got my physical well-being back after having the meridians activated (Chinese massage). Now I feel great again." [T113]

... there is still the physiological barrier "scar", the visible scar and possible troubles resulting from adhesions ...

"Abdominal pain, numbness in the lower abdomen" [T079]

"I had extreme backache due to wrong posture, wanting to go easy on the scar – physiotherapy" [T039]

... to mention just a couple.

Most Caesarean mothers are not aware of the Caesarean scar possibly being the reason for backaches or migraines. There has been too little research and education on this so far. Therefore, it is important to identify the Caesarean scar as a disruption of the healthy body and if necessary have it treated.

Furthermore, there appears to be a connection between the condition of the Caesarean scar and its acceptance by the Caesarean mother. Spontaneously, without being asked (!) many mothers told us independently, during the photo shoot, that since participating in the photo book their Caesarean scar is less disturbing, less noticeable, clearly lighter, less bulging and the photographer would have to make an effort to get a proper picture...

Back then we were surprised to hear such statements and were not really able to relate to them. In the meantime, we have realised that the "mind of the scar" also has to play a role in healing – as one mother described:

"The first Caesarean scar hurt for more than six months until I became aware of how unhappy I was about the Caesarean section, then it got better. But it was always extremely bulging and very red. I did not want to touch it and therefore did not really massage the scar to try and improve it. With the 2nd Caesarean the scar was remodeled and is now relatively nice. Possibly because the 2nd Caesarean freed me from my traumatic experience, to a large extent, which is rather strange as I was also very sad about this one and desperately wanted to deliver spontaneously." [T055]

The Caesarean section: Traumatic? (4.29)

About 42 % of the women reported having experienced the 1st Caesarean section as traumatic. With the 2nd Caesarean it was 27 % and with the 3rd 24 %.

The fact that a clear connection exists between traumatic perception and inadequate education shows that detailed preoccupation, especially early enough, with the topic of abdominal delivery is a significant part of the successful recovery from a Caesarean section.

Women from the "educated" Caesarean group experiencing the Caesarean section as traumatic occurred distinctively less frequently (7 %) compared to those uninformed women for whom this birth mostly "happened" (35 %). In other words: The risk of experiencing the Caesarean birth as traumatic is five times higher with those women not informed in time about the subject!

In practice this means that as early as the preventative medical checkups in early pregnancy – and especially in the antenatal class! – the topic "Caesarean section" should be addressed intensively. Not to stoke fears, but to prevent traumatic experiences in good time. Furthermore, the objective and comprehensive study of the section has the benefit of disproving unrealistic expectations (e.g. being painless) and revealing the attractiveness – often promoted by the media – of the Caesarean birth, often assumed to be easier, as a one-sided view.

"Adverse effects" of substantiated education regarding the Caesarean section cannot be found in our data. Therefore, there is no reason for depriving women of the detailed facts and possible consequences.

The Caesarean section: Ideal way of giving birth or harmful to health? (5.1, 6.2, 6.3)

Only for a small percentage of the women was the Caesarean section the "ideal way of giving birth": Just 16 % are of this opinion. In the group of women with an elective Caesarean section the percentage was 57 %.

One question was answered with "no" by all the women – namely, whether Caesarean section should generally replace vaginal birth in future.

This is not surprising considering that a Caesarean section is major abdominal surgery and that one in three of the Caesarean mothers had health problems afterwards.

What to do when you are afraid of birth?

The "fear of birth" is the main motive for medically unnecessary Caesareans, if you believe the obstetricians whom we interviewed. On the previous pages you have already read about some after-effects of the Caesarean section; you will see further diverse experiences with Caesarean sections in the following photographic part of the mothers.

Should you be afraid of natural birth yourself and therefore consider a Caesarean section we recommend you contact an experienced midwife. Even for women who have already successfully delivered spontaneously this can reduce existing fear and help you judge expectations of a natural birth realistically.

Be that as it may this book can educate you when preparing for a (Caesarean) birth and, thereby, be of help.

60 Caesarean mothers in
words and photographs

At a glance: Page layout and captions for the photographic part

[Number of participant]
Each woman's individual topic

Number of the participant
as well as of the photograph
used/number of picture
(separated by underscore)

Length and further
information regarding
Caesarean scar

Caption: The mother's age at the time of participation in the project and chronology of the births.
Example of abbreviations used:

V [29, g]	Vaginal delivery at the age of 29, girl
S:SPA [33, b]	Section with spinal anaesthesia at the age of 33, boy
S:EPA+GA [36, g]	Section with epidural anaesthesia and subsequent general anaesthesia at the age of 36, girl

Twins are marked as such.
Deceased children symbolised as follows (†) after the gender.

Caesarean mothers with one section

[T031]   A "lifeless" birth:

As I could not give birth by pushing contractions.

Occupation: Housewife and mother.

When I hear the word "Caesarean section" the following words come to mind spontaneously: Large abdominal operation, no "normal" birth, limited number of children (only 3 Caesareans possible), life-long scar.

I dealt with Caesareans intensively prior to my Caesarean: No.

The birth of my child (section): Natural contractions: Approx. 25 hours. Induced labour: No. Head circumference 36 cm, height 54 cm, weight 3650 g, duration of pregnancy: 41 weeks +2 days. I actually wanted to have a home birth, but 25 hours after my waters broke the cervix stopped dilating at 7 cm. The midwife sent me to hospital where I immediately received an epidural. After a further 7 hours of waiting – I desperately wanted to deliver normally – it had to be a Caesarean. It turned out that my pelvis is too narrow and I would probably never be able to give birth normally. I am missing the most beautiful part of childbirth: the experience of pushing out my child and feeling the naked, warm skin of the little one on my tummy straight after birth!!!

The indication for my section: Failure to progress during the first stage of labour.

Prior to the Caesarean I received drugs: I think contraction blockers or medication to speed up labour?

The very first eye-contact with my child: During the operation.

The first intensive physical contact with my child: Approx. 1 1/2 hours after the operation.

The Caesarean interfered with the mother-child bonding: The child was not placed on my tummy totally naked and unwashed right after birth. I miss this first and very intensive physical contact terribly!

I ascribe the following peculiarities of my child to the Caesarean birth: Namely he had two choking fits in the first two months.

I would have preferred a natural (vaginal) birth: Yes.

I feel inferior due to having missed out on the experience of birth: Yes.

A Caesarean birth possibly has negative effects on the child: If the Caesarean takes place abruptly the child is not prepared for birth, it might not start breathing immediately. Furthermore, heart and circulation are not particularly stimulated because the child is not pressed through the narrow birth canal.

Due to the following the rate of Caesareans is rising: Physicians are paid more for a Caesarean section (?) and it does not require as much time as a normal birth. And physicians and/or midwives suggest a Caesarean more often and a woman who is going through the worst of pains is open to anything that will stop the pain, i.e. they agree to a Caesarean easier while having labour pains!

My fundamental attitude on the topic "Caesarean": In case of emergency I am glad that the Caesarean exists! But in all other cases I find the Caesarean unnecessary since a woman thereby misses the most beautiful thing in the world, bringing her own child into the world through her own strength and having it placed onto her tummy immediately after. Besides nobody talks about the days after the Caesarean where you cannot get up to care for your child (change nappies, bath, ...).

My Caesarean scar (length approx. 14 cm):

My partner does not like touching it.
A light crooked line, bending outwards slightly.

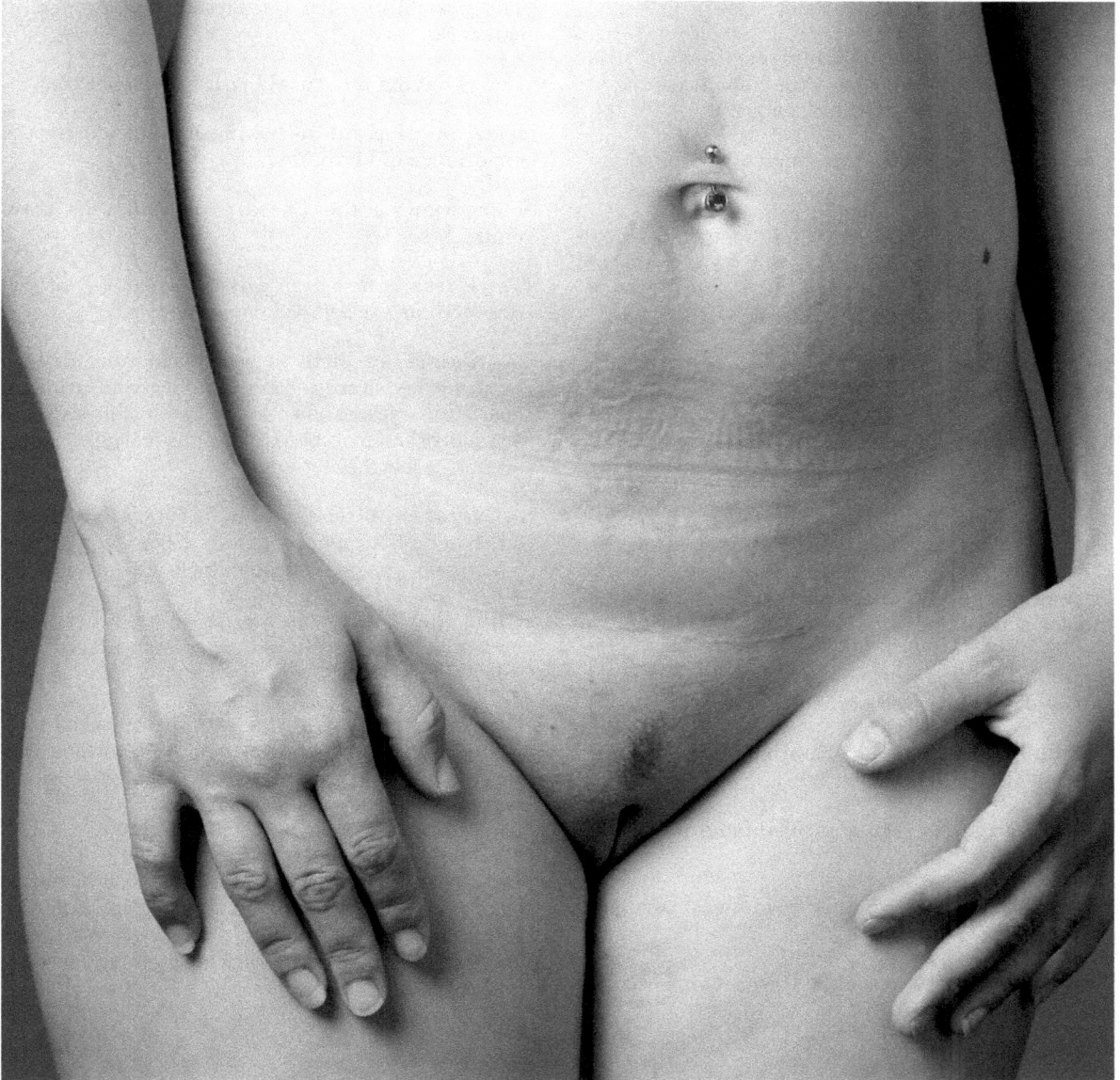

[T129]   We caught up on everything:

A very empathetic midwife stood by us in the first hours.

Occupation: Registered paediatric nurse.

When I hear the word "Caesarean section" the following words come to mind spontaneously: Scar, baby, pain, anaesthesia, separation.

I dealt with Caesareans intensively prior to my Caesarean: No.

The birth of my child (section): Contractions: No. Head circumference 32 cm, height 48 cm, weight 2460 g. Emergency caesarean section in the 38th week due to preeclampsia/HELLP syndrome.

Prior to the Caesarean I received drugs: Antihypertensive drugs.

The very first eye-contact and intensive physical contact with my child: Approx. 2 hours after the operation.

The following complications occurred after the Caesarean: Approx. 4 cm open suture during redressing was stitched up under local anaesthesia – the evening of the same day.

I suffered from depression after the Caesarean: I cried a lot, asked myself why.

My child had serious health problems / has serious health problems now: No.

I would have preferred a natural (vaginal) birth: Yes.

I was afraid of pain during birth/of perineal trauma: No.

I was afraid of a possible Caesarean section: Yes.

The possibility of a Caesarean was prognosticated: No.

I miss having a natural birth experience: Yes

I feel inferior due to having missed out on the experience of birth: Yes.

I experienced the Caesarean section as traumatic: Yes.

The Caesarean section was the ideal way of giving birth as far as I am concerned: No.

My Caesarean birth is seen as a fully-fledged birth by my family, friends and acquaintances: Apart from a few acquaintances, when girlfriends talk about their "normal" births I have the feeling of not being able to join the conversation.

A Caesarean birth possibly has negative effects on the child: It cannot get ready (before term), it gets cold – loud – bright – uncomfortable way too fast.

I find that Caesarean section is trivialised and minimised by the media (newspaper, magazines, television, ...): Yes.

Due to the following the rate of Caesareans is rising: High number of problematic pregnancies; possibility of elective Caesarean section; maybe economic reasons on the part of the hospital.

My fundamental attitude on the topic "Caesarean": Clearly, health of mother and child have first priority! I was totally prepared for a vaginal birth, was surprised by the section and do not wish this experience on any other woman (which I know is impossible – nevertheless).

My Caesarean scar (length approx. 15 cm):

Clearly visible; I find it very long; it is still red – hope it will fade someday.
Due to another surgical suture on my abdomen it is even harder for me to
accept my Caesarean scar. I feel a dragging pain around my Caesarean
scar with weather changes, numb feeling around the scar.

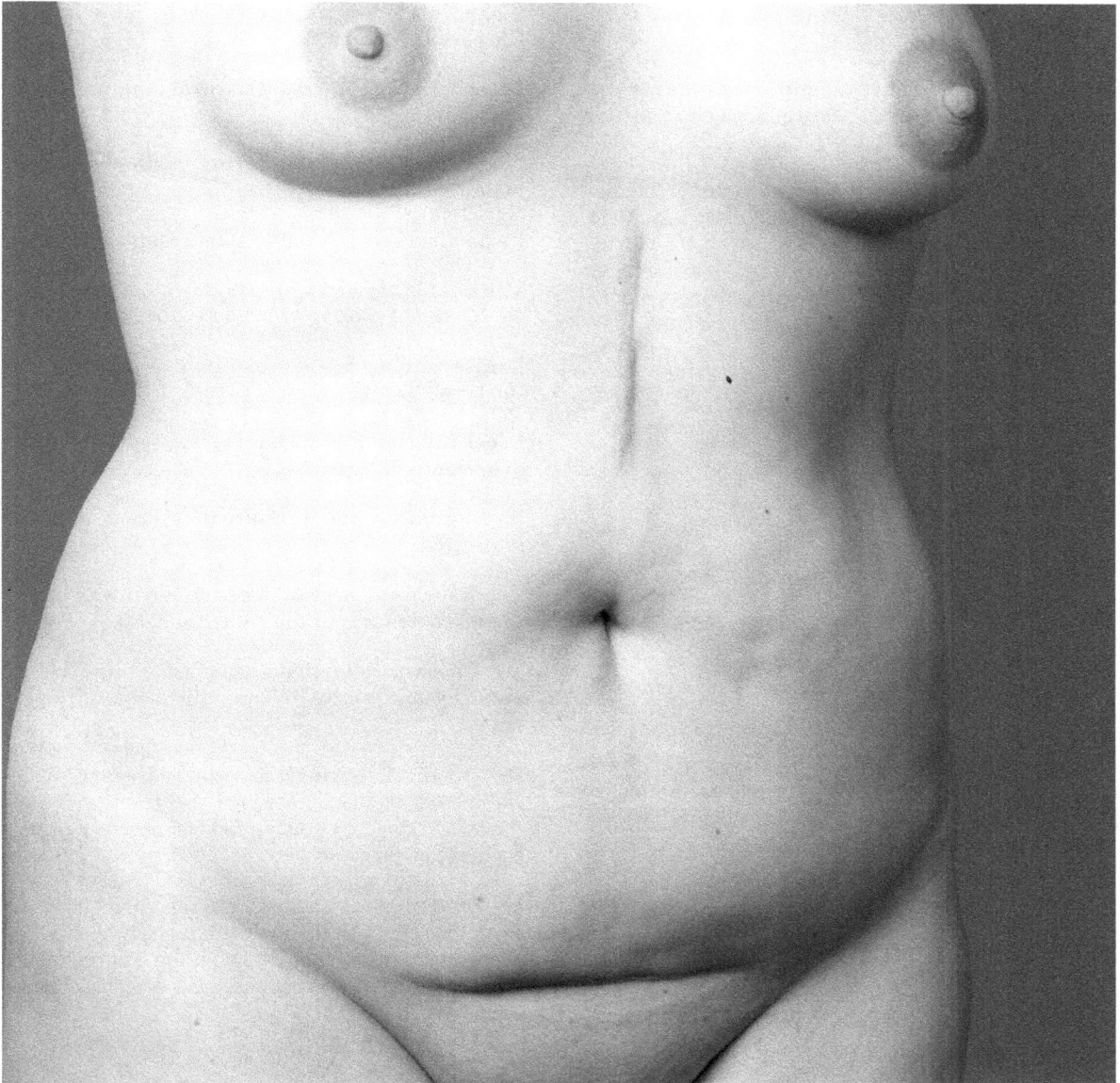

I always thought that a Caesarean would not affect me... only others.

Occupation: Teacher.

When I hear the word "Caesarean section" the following words come to mind spontaneously: Unexpected, inescapable, being at someone's mercy, rescue, pain.

The birth of my child (section): Natural contractions: Approx. 20 hours. Induced labour: Drip, duration unknown. Head circumference 33 cm, height 49 cm, weight 2825 g, duration of pregnancy: 38 weeks. 2 ½ weeks too early, 26 hours in the delivery room, cervix wouldn't dilate, therefore epidural, cervix dilated, then inadequate contractions – only chance for my daughter to be born: Caesarean section.

The indication for my section: Failure to progress at pelvic floor, uterine insufficiency.

The following complications occurred during the Caesarean: Epidural was renewed for the operation, was not 100 % effective. During the operation (after the section) I felt the surgery and received a general anaesthesia immediately.

The very first eye-contact and intensive physical contact with my child: Approx. 1 hour after the operation.

I had difficulties breastfeeding after the Caesarean: Engorgement of the breasts only on the fourth day. Breastfeeding was or is only possible with nipple shields. I am still breastfeeding.

The Caesarean did not interfere with the mother-child bonding: I have no comparison but when I saw my daughter for the first time I knew that I would do anything for her and that I adore her.

I suffered from depression after the Caesarean: No.

I have been having health problems since my Caesarean section: Migraines.

I would have preferred a natural (vaginal) birth: Yes.

I was afraid of pain during birth/of perineal trauma: No.

I was afraid of a possible Caesarean section: No.

The possibility of a Caesarean was prognosticated: Not during pregnancy but during birth.

I miss having a natural birth experience: The "first cry".

I feel inferior due to having missed out on the experience of birth: No.

I experienced the Caesarean section as traumatic: No.

The Caesarean section was the ideal way of giving birth as far as I am concerned: No.

My Caesarean birth is seen as a fully-fledged birth by my family, friends and acquaintances: Yes.

Due to the following the rate of Caesareans is rising: A lot of people may think that it is "easier" and "faster". Taking into account famous people's births it seems to be fashionable.

My fundamental attitude on the topic "Caesarean": I am glad that there is the possibility of a Caesarean section. But it should remain the last alternative – when natural birth is not possible – after having tried everything.

My Caesarean scar (length approx. 9.5 cm):

Straight, short section. From time to time I feel a dragging pain and itching. In the first two weeks it had to be cleaned (purulent). I treat my Caesarean scar with "Bepanthen" ointment.

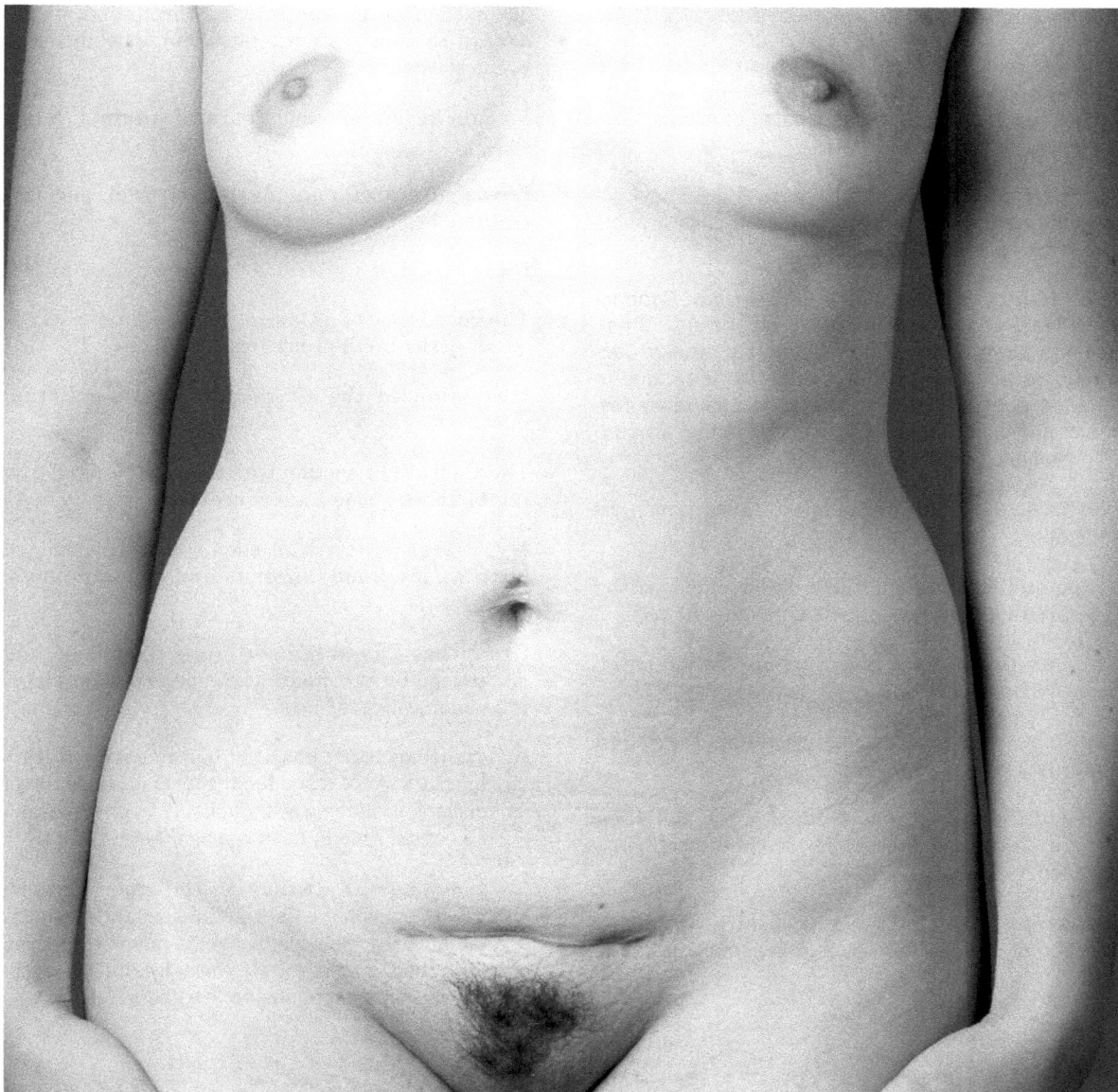

Caesarean mothers with one section

Due to the following the rate of Caesareans is rising:

Fear of pain and failure during a vaginal birth. A woman does not want to lower her guard; the Caesarean can be planned. It suits today's society!

Occupation: Head of PR & marketing.

When I hear the word "Caesarean section" the following words come to mind spontaneously: Rescue, easy, painless, breastfeeding problems, lacking feeling of happiness.

The birth of my first child (vaginal delivery): Induction due to preeclampsia, oversized child – pubic symphysis separation (extreme).

The birth of my second child (section): Contractions: No. Head circumference 35 cm, height 49 cm, weight 3000 g, duration of pregnancy: 38 weeks. Caesarean section, approx. 2 weeks before term, due to renewed pubic symphysis separation. Ultimately rescue of the child: very serious infection in the newborn – vaginal birth impossible.

The indication for my section: Pubic symphysis separation.

In the end the following persons decided on the Caesarean: Physicians, myself, physiotherapist.

The very first eye-contact with my second child: Approx. 3 hours after the operation.

The Caesarean interfered with the mother-child bonding: No.

I had difficulties breastfeeding after the Caesarean: Could only breastfeed for three months, no lactation.

My second child had serious health problems: Infection of the newborn (already prenatal); at risk of SIDS.

My second child was injured through the Caesarean section: A slight scratch on the head caused by the scalpel.

I would have preferred a natural (vaginal) birth: Yes.

I was afraid of pain during birth/of perineal trauma: No.

I was afraid of a possible Caesarean section: No.

The possibility of a Caesarean was prognosticated after the birth of my first child: Yes.

I experienced the Caesarean section as traumatic: No.

The Caesarean section was the ideal way of giving birth as far as I am concerned: No.

My Caesarean birth is seen as a fully-fledged birth by my family, friends and acquaintances: Yes.

I find that Caesarean section is trivialised and minimised by the media (newspaper, magazines, television, ...): Yes.

A Caesarean birth possibly has negative effects on the child: All of a sudden the child is pulled out of its familiar surrounding, without using its own strength – does not necessarily have lasting effects.

My fundamental attitude on the topic "Caesarean": In my opinion the Caesarean is a great possibility or alternative if it's impossible for the mother to deliver, or for the child to be delivered, vaginally! But it is an operation which should not be done without indication!

My Caesarean scar (length approx. 9 cm):

It is shaped like a "smiley". I do not feel my Caesarean scar. It healed
without any problems. It is easy for me to accept my Caesarean scar.

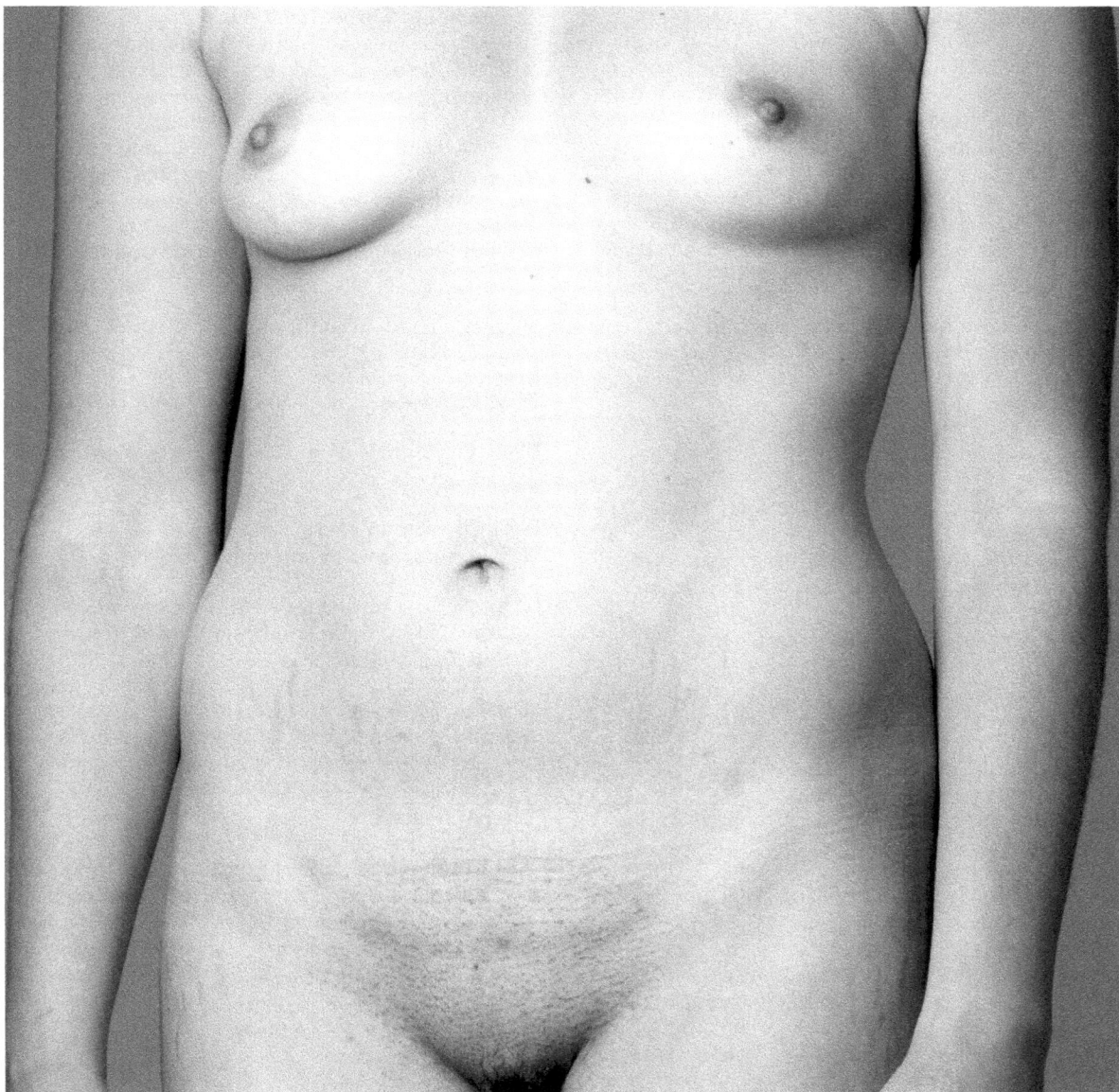

Caesarean mothers with one section

[T 117] The Caesarean interfered with the mother-child bonding:

More bonding with both my older children than with my Caesarean child:
you should not lift them, they are not allowed to be so rough etc.

Occupation: Forwarding merchant.

When I hear the word "Caesarean section" the following words come to mind spontaneously: Pain, child and mother at risk, fashionable (elective Caesarean section), restricted physical resilience, jealousy (siblings).

The birth of my first child (vaginal delivery): "Normal" duration of 10 ½ hours. Strenuous but wonderful.

The birth of my second child (vaginal delivery): Personally this delivery went too quickly for me (2 ½ hours).

I dealt with Caesareans intensively prior to my first Caesarean: No.

The birth of my third child (section): Natural contractions: Approx. 2 ½ hours. Head circumference 36 cm, height 54 cm, weight 3980 g, duration of pregnancy: 40 weeks. The Caesarean was decided on as I had fever and very strong contractions. Heart rate was double the normal, it was very stressful.

The indication for my section: Pathological CTG, fever sub partu.

Prior to the Caesarean, I received drugs: No.

The Caesarean proceeded without complications: Yes.

The very first eye-contact with my third child: Approx. 1 ½ hours after the operation.

The first intensive physical contact with my third child: Approx. 7 hours after the operation.

I suffered from depression after the Caesarean: No.

I was able to breastfeed without difficulty after the Caesarean: I did, however, constantly have to advise the nurse in the children's medical unit, otherwise she would have given supplementary feeding.

I have been having health problems since my Caesarean section: For a very long time I did not have or I have not got my bladder under control.

I would have preferred a natural (vaginal) birth: Yes.

I was afraid of pain during birth/of perineal trauma: No.

I was afraid of a possible Caesarean section: No.

The possibility of a Caesarean was prognosticated: No.

The Caesarean section was the ideal way of giving birth as far as I am concerned: No.

I find that Caesarean section is trivialised and minimised by the media (newspaper, magazines, television, ...): Yes.

Due to the following the rate of Caesareans is rising: Fear of birth pain, exaggerated precaution, low faith in the natural way of birth, pipe dreams of a painless birth, media reports. Belief in being slim faster after a Caesarean.

My fundamental attitude on the topic "Caesarean": In the case of medical reasons the Caesarean should not be questioned. But definitely for reasons of convenience, one could be disappointed. I would understand anxiety as being a reason for a Caesarean, but only if already experienced. Fundamentally I am against elective Caesarean sections.

My Caesarean scar (length approx. 18 cm):

I find my Caesarean scar ugly. From time to time – mostly when the weather changes – I feel a dragging pain. Around the site of the section I have very little or no feeling and it has a raised, uneven feel to it.

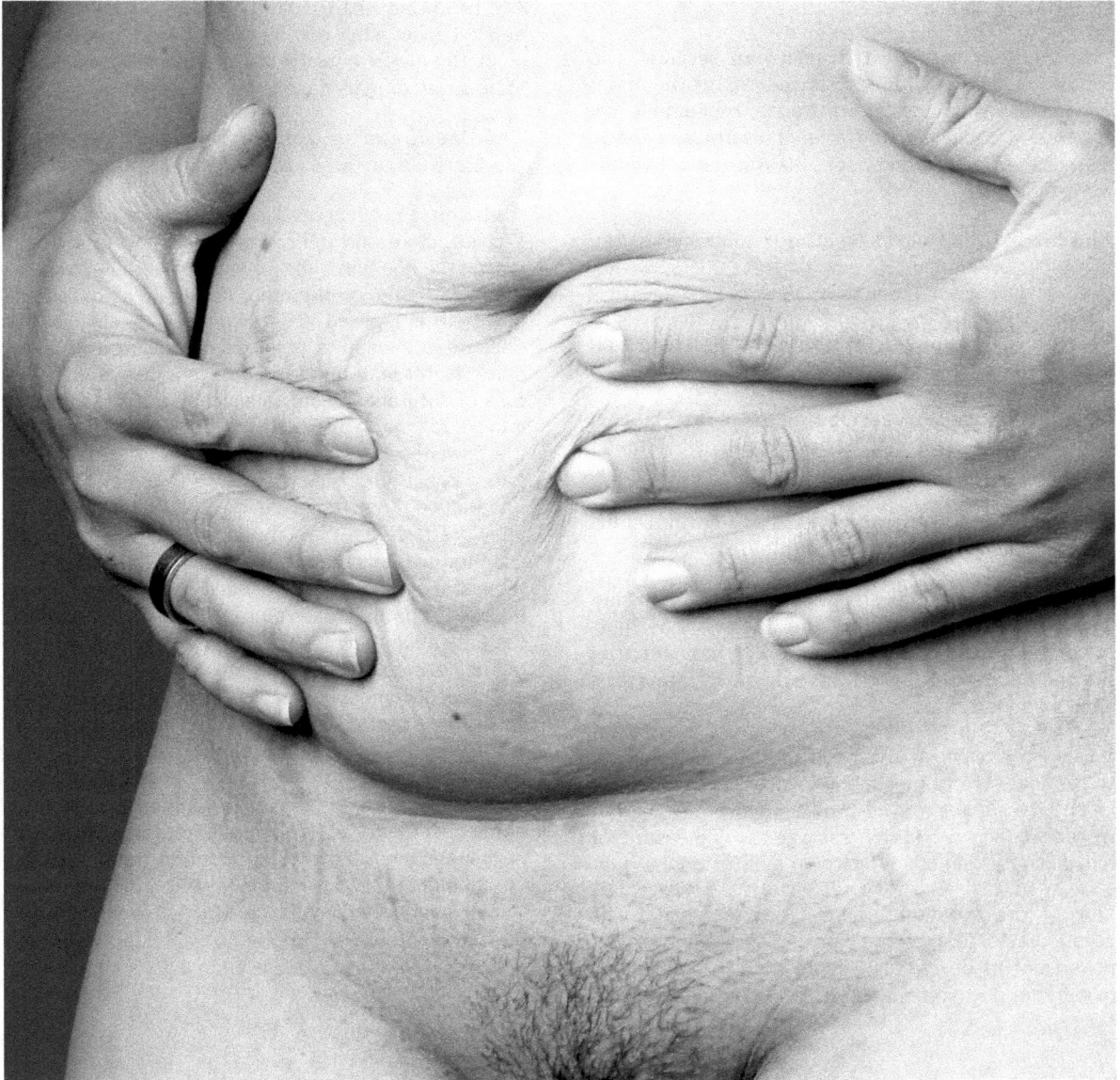

Caesarean mothers with one section

His first cry made me forget everything:

That I was lying, cut open, in a large bright room was secondary.

Occupation: Office worker.

When I hear the word "Caesarean section" the following words come to mind spontaneously: Becoming a mother, state of trance, excitement, impatience (I could not wait after the term was fixed), softness (it was somehow soft, the way the physicians worked on me).

The birth of my child (section): Contractions: No. Head circumference 35 cm, height 50 cm, weight 3060 g, duration of pregnancy: 38 weeks +6 days.

The indication for my section: Breech presentation (and this with the first pregnancy).

I had difficulties breastfeeding after the Caesarean: Yes and no, my nipples were too sensitive therefore I expressed for 4 months.

The very first eye-contact with my child: During the operation.

The first intensive physical contact with my child: Approx. 2 hours after the operation. My husband and my son could have been with me right after the operation, unfortunately an emergency Caesarean section interfered.

I ascribe the following peculiarities of my child to the Caesarean birth: My son always used to smile when clothing was pulled over his head or he had to wear a woollen hat. I think this was not unpleasant for him since he did not go through the birth canal.

Due to the following the rate of Caesareans is rising: Faster for the physician, generally controllable, risks want to be reduced, more medical indications (e.g. better nutrition = larger children), more complications.

My fundamental attitude on the topic "Caesarean": It is definitely not the natural way of delivering a child. But luckily a justifiable alternative when life has to be saved or risks need to be minimised.

The Caesarean section was the ideal way of giving birth as far as I am concerned: Yes.

Additional notes: I dealt with both ways of delivering a child before and during my pregnancy. In my opinion, on the one hand, the Caesarean birth is trivialised these days and, on the other hand, the so-called normal birth is idolised. Often women are told that the Caesarean section is painless, trouble-free and very quick. Not true. It hurts too, just in a different way. Or fans of natural birth broadcast that one can only turn into a super mum after going through the pain of birth, the powerlessness, the ecstasy. Also not true. Therefore it is not surprising that these women do not feel understood. That they develop a sense of inferiority. They are forsaken by both sides. Only the ones who went through this themselves know what it is like [...] I think that a woman does not become a mother through the pain of birth. It takes more. The will to have a child, the time of carrying the wonder in one's body and last but not least the time after – the way in which one raises the child, what you instill in the child for life. In my case it was not necessary to do a Caesarean section but advisable. I would not have had to do it. But what for? Just to proudly be able to say I have given birth to a breech baby? Am I more of a mother then? As far as I am concerned: No! I do not understand why I should have taken a risk if everything went fine for 9 months. I am thankful that I have a healthy baby. 200 years ago I would not have had a choice. Maybe everything would have worked out well. Maybe not. P.S.: I am especially delighted when men discuss and judge this topic.

My Caesarean scar (length approx. 14 cm):

In the beginning I was afraid the scar could open up. The nurses tried to calm me down [...]. Anyhow, I moved very cautiously in the beginning. [...] The scar healed beautifully, fast and without a problem. Its shape is like a smile.

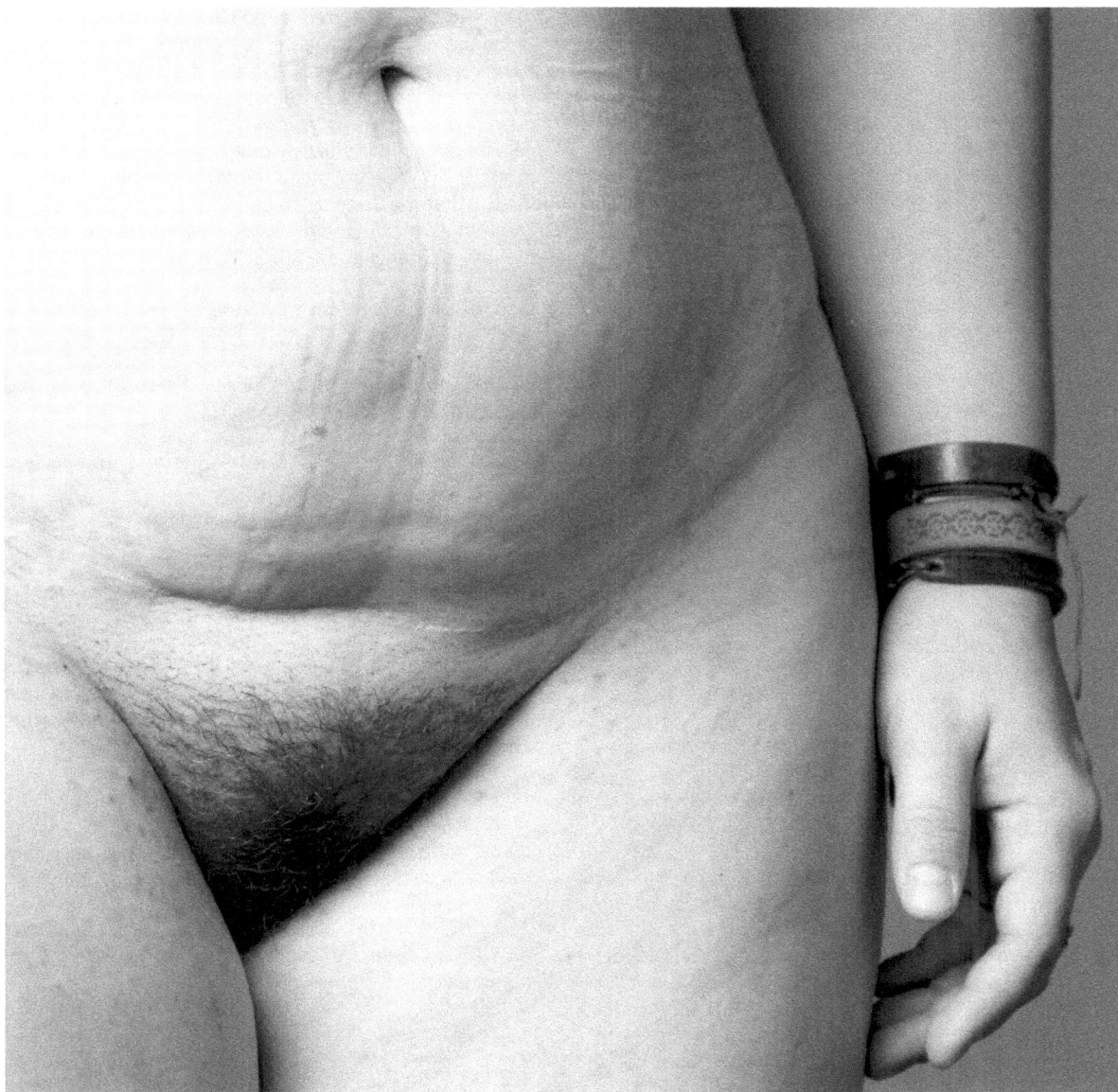

[T066] I spent time contemplating the Caesarean section prior to my Caesarean birth:

Because I was afraid of it and did not ever want to experience "something like that".

Occupation: Bank clerk on maternity leave.

When I hear the word "Caesarean section" the following words come to mind spontaneously: "Emergency exit for the baby", my scars: Abdomen + soul, sadness because I miss having a birth experience, fortunate that I had the possibility and my little one was delivered healthy, pain.

The birth of my first child (vaginal delivery): After 18 hours of contractions luckily without a Caesarean section. A little complicated – but the most beautiful and exhilarating experience ever.

The birth of my second child (section): Natural contractions: Yes, duration unknown. Induced labour: Approx. 8 hours. Head circumference 35 cm, height 52 cm, weight 3120 g duration of pregnancy: 40 weeks. Wrong lie, umbilical cord around the neck, bad heart tones, placental abruption – Caesarean section. Very fortunate, daughter healthy. Great sadness: I miss the rush of joy.

The indication for my section: Transverse lie, extension of the neck, umbilical cord around the neck – bad heart tones and ultimately placental abruption.

The very first eye-contact with my second child: During the operation.

The first intensive physical contact with my second child: Approx. 30 minutes after the operation.

I was able to breastfeed without difficulty after the Caesarean: I breastfed for 7 months.

The Caesarean did not interfere with the mother-child bonding in the long term: But I observed that my daughter was very fearful and agitated. In the first hours I only held her on my tummy. And a few weeks in

bed with me, wanted to let go slowly. And I think it was good that way. My daughter is a cheerful, even-tempered baby. She slept through from the beginning and is just very happy. The extreme difference to my firstborn who was so happy right after birth was very noticeable. My daughter immediately cried when I just lifted her from one breast to the other. The paediatrician conceded that the Caesarean as well as the complications in pregnancy affected my daughter. She had to fight for her life so many times. She was just afraid.

I would have preferred a natural (vaginal) birth: Yes.

I was afraid of pain during birth/of perineal trauma: No.

I was afraid of a possible Caesarean section: Yes.

I miss having a natural birth experience: Yes

The Caesarean section was the ideal way of giving birth as far as I am concerned: No.

A Caesarean birth possibly has negative effects on the child: But as a mother you can compensate a lot. I find elective Caesarean sections terrible because babies are "pulled out" totally unprepared.

Due to the following the rate of Caesareans is rising: Mothers are afraid of pain during birth or injuries and that they won't have "great sex" anymore, private physicians fulfilling the request, scheduling.

My fundamental attitude on the topic "Caesarean": The Caesarean section should remain an "emergency exit".

My Caesarean scar (length approx. 11.5 cm):

I hardly ever feel my Caesarean scar, only e.g. in winter before heavy snowfall. In the beginning I treated it with "Enercetica" lotion. Scar treatment with acupuncture massage.

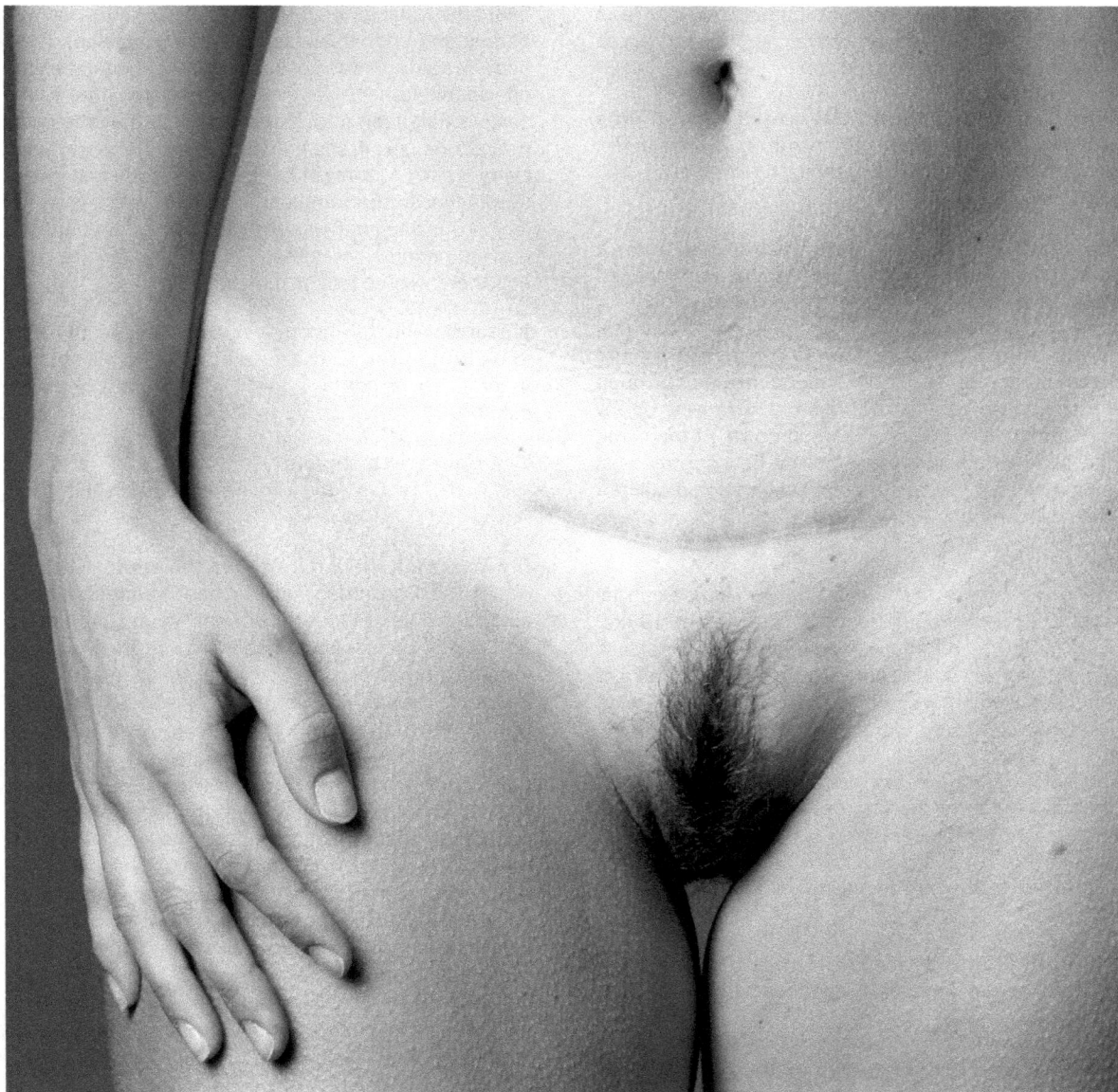

[T013]   Physically I felt a lot better after the Caesarean than after my first, vaginal delivery:

I was able to care for my child a lot better!

Occupation: At the moment fulltime mother and housewife, family manager. I have completed a degree in vocal performance (Mozarteum).

When I hear the word "Caesarean section" the following words come to mind spontaneously: (My) scar, my daughter, operating theatre, birth, epidural.

The birth of my first child (vaginal delivery): Because of gestational diabetes labour was induced three days before term. I lay in the delivery room for three whole days with 30 hours of contractions [...]. HORROR! My son weighed 3920 g and had a head circumference of 38 cm. My perineum was cut open and two midwives plus my husband were lying on my huge tummy and pressing our son down. At the same time two obstetricians were pulling between my legs using a vacuum extractor. Weeks later I could still not sit or walk properly without pain. Back then I swore to myself: "Never again!"

The birth of my second child (section): Contractions: No. Head circumference 36 cm, height 49 cm, weight 3280 g, duration of pregnancy: 38 weeks. A dream! After my son's "horror birth" it could only get better – everything was planned, the pain that followed was a joke compared to the pain of the first delivery.

The indication for my section: The referral said "birth trauma after the first delivery" plus gestational diabetes and streptococcus.

I suffered from depression after the Caesarean: No.

I was able to breastfeed without difficulty after the Caesarean: I am still breastfeeding.

My second child had serious health problems: When our daughter was born I already noticed i.e.

heard her rattling, coughing, gasping. [...] After she was bathed and undressed (according to my husband) the midwife said she was not sure but she thought the little one should rather be put into an incubator. After all the devices had been attached it was clear that she could not get enough air, she then also started wheezing with every breath. An x-ray of her lung was made and, thereby, diagnosed that amniotic fluid had collected in her lungs. Our daughter was treated with an antibiotic (to prevent pneumonia) in the neonatal unit for one week and there was no lasting damage.

I ascribe the following peculiarities of my second child to the Caesarean birth: She will not take a comforter or bottle – only my breast, searching for comfort.

The Caesarean section was the ideal way of giving birth as far as I am concerned: In this case: yes.

My fundamental attitude on the topic "Caesarean": The Caesarean section has definitely already saved the lives of thousands of babies and/or mothers and is well on its way to becoming the most modern form of "normal delivery". Anyhow we should not stab nature in the back out of pure selfishness. Should a woman have difficulties in pregnancy, with the child and/or her own body or also massive psychological problems – even if there is just the smallest indication, not just simulated – then I find it good if an elective Caesarean section can help these women, as in my case. [...] However, I do not understand women, like some stars & starlets, who choose to have a Caesarean section because of their timetable or the wrong ideal of beauty. Should I conceive a third time [...] and have gestational diabetes once again, I would definitely have a Caesarean section again. In a pregnancy without gestational diabetes I would favour a spontaneous vaginal delivery.

My Caesarean scar (length approx. 17 cm):

It itches sometimes. Every time I shower, bath, get dressed, shave or apply lotion I am reminded of my daughter's birth – my dream child with a dream birth. The scar is part of me like my hands and feet!

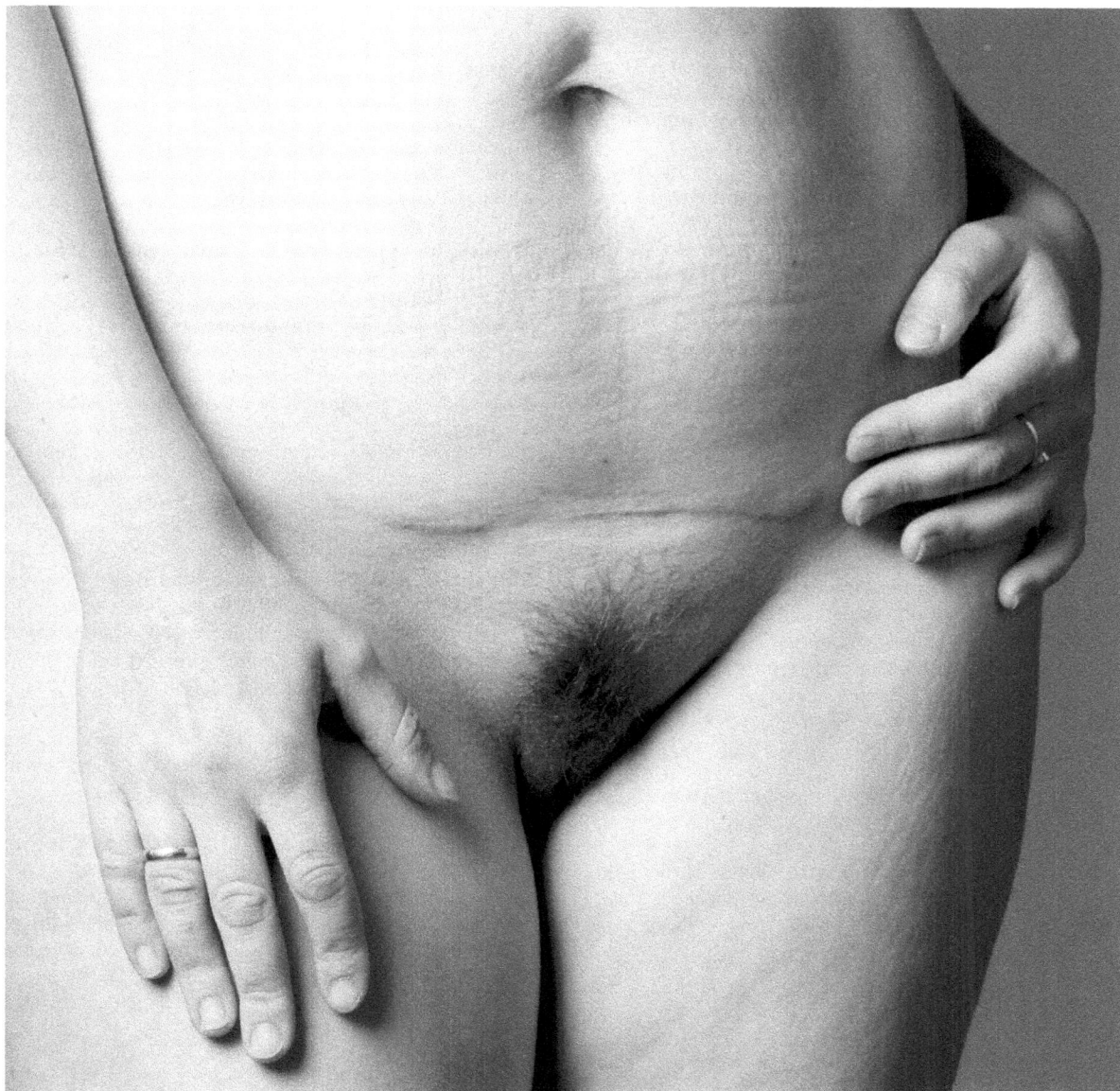

[T052] A Caesarean birth possibly has negative effects on the child:

Well... neither yes nor no! The child does not have to fight or work for anything – it does not have to go through anything: Effects on the personality!!!

Occupation: Physiotherapist.

When I hear the word "Caesarean section" the following words come to mind spontaneously: Oh dear! Thank God, scar, pain, hopefully a "normal birth" with the second child.

I dealt with Caesareans intensively prior to my Caesarean: No.

The birth of my first child (section): Natural contractions: Approx. 11 hours. Induced labour: Approx. 3 hours drip. Head circumference 37 ½ cm, height 53 cm, weight 3880 g, duration of pregnancy: 41 weeks +3 days. 10 days beyond - enema - labour onset - 6 hours of strong contractions - 3 hours drip - bad heart tones - no cervical dilatation - emergency Caesarean section.

The indication for my Caesarean section: My son was a so-called "stargazer", did not drop.

The following complications occurred during the Caesarean: Spinal anaesthesia; extreme sharp pain caused by the anaesthetic spreading between the shoulder blades, slight shortage of breath, nausea.

The very first eye-contact with my first child: During the operation.

The first intensive physical contact with my first child: Approx. 1 hour after the operation.

The Caesarean interfered with the mother-child bonding: In the beginning I could not carry my child, bath him or change nappies. The first contact was with my husband - our son (three years old now) is a REAL!!! daddy's boy.

I had difficulties breastfeeding after the Caesarean: I had problems with the left nipple; approx. 8 breast infections in total. I breastfed for more than 1 year.

I ascribe the following peculiarities of my first child to the Caesarean birth: Fine motor skills slow and very, very lazy in the first year.

I would have preferred a natural (vaginal) birth: Yes.

I was afraid of pain during birth/of perineal trauma: No.

I was afraid of a possible Caesarean section: No.

I miss having a natural birth experience: Yes.

I experienced the Caesarean section as traumatic: Yes.

The birth of my second child (vaginal delivery): Very, very long and difficult birth! 10 days beyond term - induction - 10 hours of contractions - cervix won't dilate, epidural - cervix dilated after 20 hours - forceps - but without Caesarean section!

Due to the following the rate of Caesareans is rising: Fear of contractions or complications, modern, happens quickly - date can be planned exactly.

My fundamental attitude on the topic "Caesarean": I feel sorry for every woman who needs a Caesarean. On the other hand I am thankful to medical science that it exists, otherwise presumably a lot of mothers and babies would die at birth - as in times before the Caesarean!

My Caesarean scar (length approx. 10 cm):

Approx. six months after the section I had pain again and again. One half of
the scar is fine, the other half is rough and healed with a bulge. When I touch
it – unpleasant feeling all around. I am happy that it is so far down.

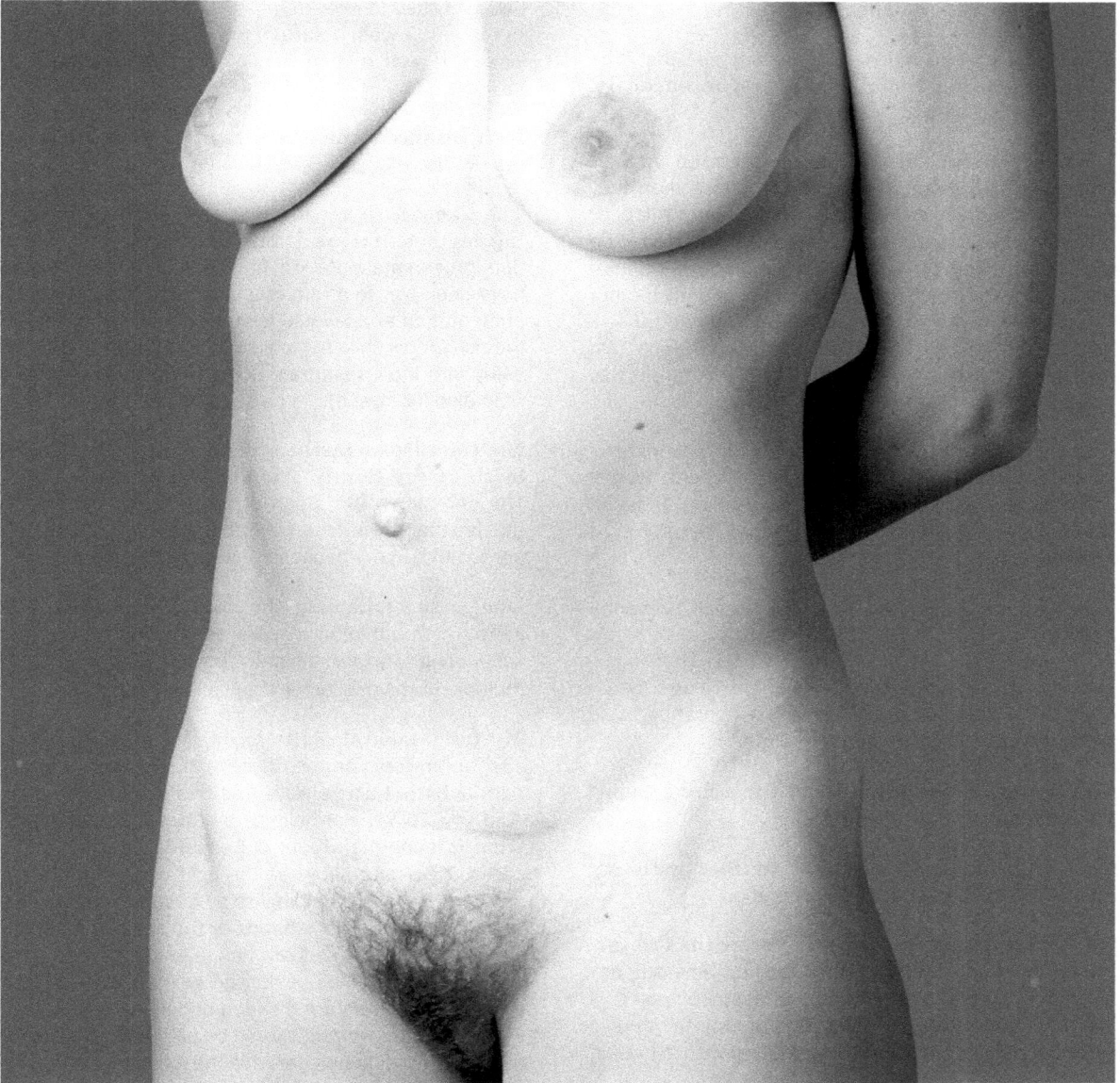

At first yes, but not at any price (because of breech presentation).

Occupation: Radiographer.

When I hear the word "Caesarean section" the following words come to mind spontaneously: Birth, baby, scar, surgery, hospital.

I was delivered by Caesarean section myself (because of breech presentation): Back then they only found out when my mother was already in labour – emergency Caesarean section. As a child I used to be afraid of my mother's Caesarean scar. A huge indentation from the navel to the pubic bone. I told my mother I would never want such a scar. She explained that it only looked that way because it had to go really fast and that the scars are made in a totally different way nowadays. That put my mind at rest.

The birth of my child (section): Contractions: No. Head circumference 36 cm, height 50 cm, weight 3100 g, duration of pregnancy: 38 weeks +1 day. It was a great experience. When I heard the first cry I cried for joy...

The indication for my section: Breech presentation.

Prior to the Caesarean, I received drugs: Sedatives (IV). I was already lying on the operating table when the anaesthetist offered it to me.

The very first eye-contact with my child: During the operation.

The first intensive physical contact with my child: Approx. 1 hour after the operation.

I had difficulties breastfeeding after the Caesarean: I could only breastfeed for the first time one day later, they "forgot" about it in the anaesthetic recovery room. He had problems latching on at first, the nurses were not very helpful and I had to deal with it myself.

I was advised to express milk – after he had got used to the teat it was, unfortunately, finally over. After two weeks he was a "bottle-child" (formula) because my milk dried up.

I experienced the Caesarean section as traumatic: No.

The Caesarean section was the ideal way of giving birth as far as I am concerned: In my situation (breech presentation, first child) definitely. I would have been way to afraid of a vaginal birth with breech presentation and I would have clenched out of fear of the risk for my child (which is not beneficial). I felt a lot safer with the Caesarean; doing the best for my child (and also for myself).

My Caesarean birth is seen as a fully-fledged birth by my family, friends and acquaintances: The only person to laugh at me was the midwife at the postnatal exercise class because I "immediately agreed to surgery because of a breech presentation".

Due to the following the rate of Caesareans is rising: Some think it may be less painful; better time scheduling (partner, holiday, care for siblings), rise in multiple births caused by artificial insemination.

My fundamental attitude on the topic "Caesarean": In my opinion the Caesarean section is a totally normal birth. I also always find this question strange: "Did you deliver normally or by Caesarean section?" What is abnormal about a Caesarean section? It is called "helping a baby see the light of day", there are different ways of "helping" e.g. forceps, vacuum extractor, gynaecologist's hands or the scalpel. An emergency Caesarean section has already saved many women's and babies' lives and women who request a Caesarean without indication should also receive it. Every pregnant woman should be allowed to decide for herself. Each one has her reasons for it.

My Caesarean scar (length approx. 15 cm):

I think my physician did a very good job: It is situated very low and therefore really only visible when I am wearing nothing at all. But I do not have and never had problems with my scar, neither physically nor psychologically. Far from it, I am even a little proud of it – because this is the way I gave birth to my son.

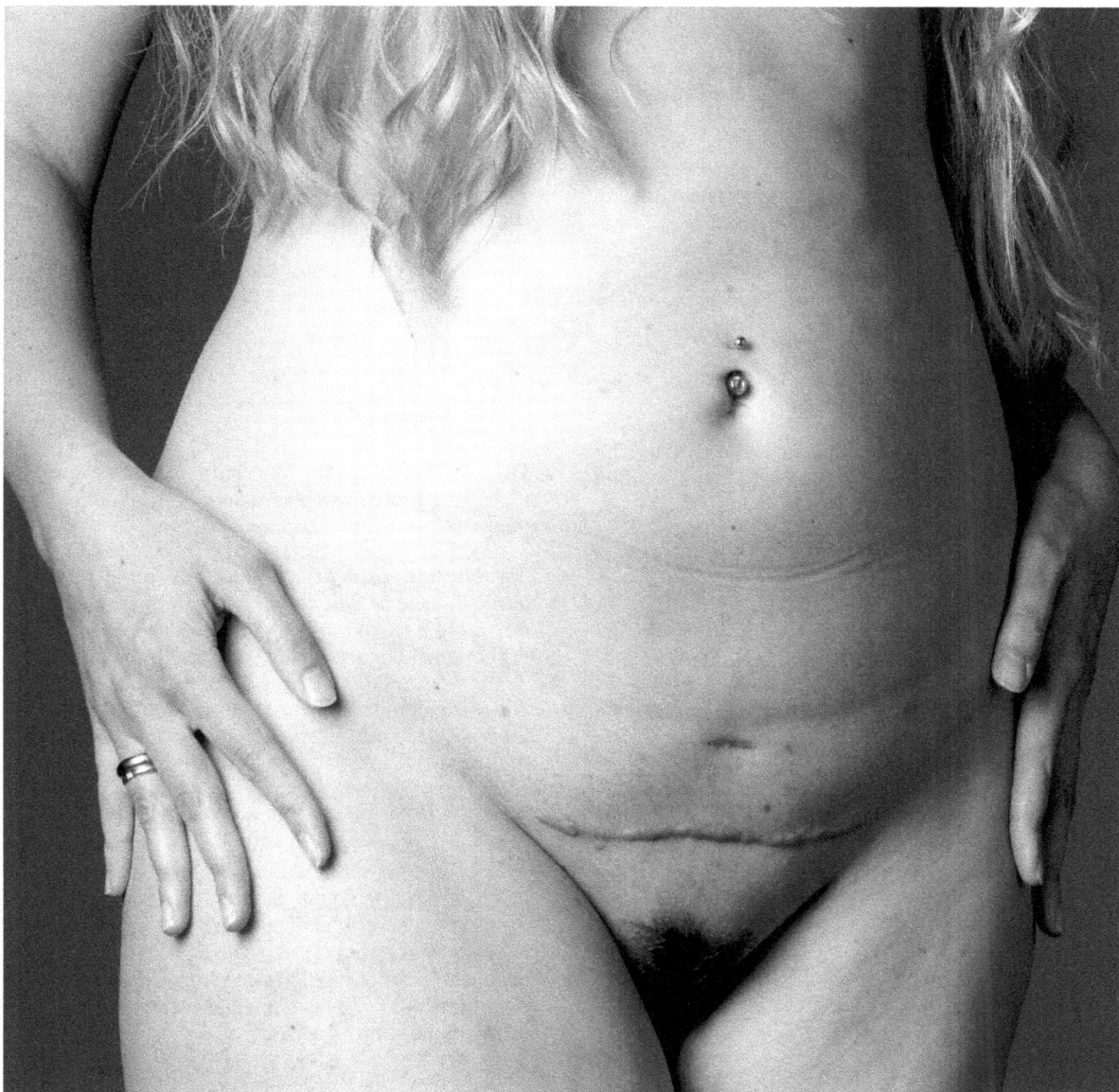

Caesarean mothers with one section

[T151] Caesarean sections did not matter to me
        before the delivery:

I was 100 % positive that I would be able to deliver vaginally.

Occupation: Physician.

When I hear the word "Caesarean section" the following words come to mind spontaneously: Why "Caesar"?, pain, paralysis.

The birth of my child (section): Natural contractions: Approx. 7 hours. Head circumference 34 cm, height 52 cm, weight 3720 g, duration of pregnancy: 40 weeks.

The indication for my section: Cephalopelvic disproportion.

Prior to the Caesarean, I received drugs: Antibiotic due to rupture of membranes.

The following complications occurred during the Caesarean: Shortness of breath and nausea when being sutured.

The very first eye-contact with my child: During the operation.

The first intensive physical contact with my child: Approx. 45 minutes after the operation.

The Caesarean interfered with the mother-child bonding: Mother-child contact so much later!!!

I ascribe the following peculiarities of my child to the Caesarean birth: Beautiful head shape; does not appear squashed when compared to other babies.

I had health problems after my Caesarean: Four weeks of pain.

I would have preferred a natural (vaginal) birth: Yes.

I was afraid of pain during birth/of perineal trauma: No.

I was afraid of a possible Caesarean section: No.

I miss having a natural birth experience: Yes.

The Caesarean gives me the feeling of not having done everything for my child: Yes.

A Caesarean birth possibly has negative effects on the child: Difficulties adapting initially – too fast, too cold.

The Caesarean section is trivialised and minimised by the media (newspaper, magazines, television, …): Yes!!

Due to the following the rate of Caesareans is rising: Reduced capacity for suffering (fear of contractions), bad education and trivialisation!!

My fundamental attitude on the topic "Caesarean": In case of emergency, for a baby's well-being – otherwise never. I think an elective Caesarean section is short-sighted, unenlightened, trivialised.

Additional notes: "Caesarean section" – what a pathetic expression – because emperors were delivered that way. And what about the mothers? How many do you think survived this mostly underestimated abdominal surgery? A proper abdominal suture, a sterile operation, septic treatment – all of this was not available – so it could not have been a lot… Thanks to my adrenalin level and the euphoria about my daughter most of my symptoms were "concealed" or only registered a lot later. I think the section is trivialised because this is the case with a lot of mothers. You forget negative things a lot faster than positive ones – which is the child. It compensates for everything.

My Caesarean scar (length approx. 15 cm):

In the beginning I often used to observe the scar disbelievingly in the mirror –
as if it was not a part of me. Now, more than a year later, I can accept it.

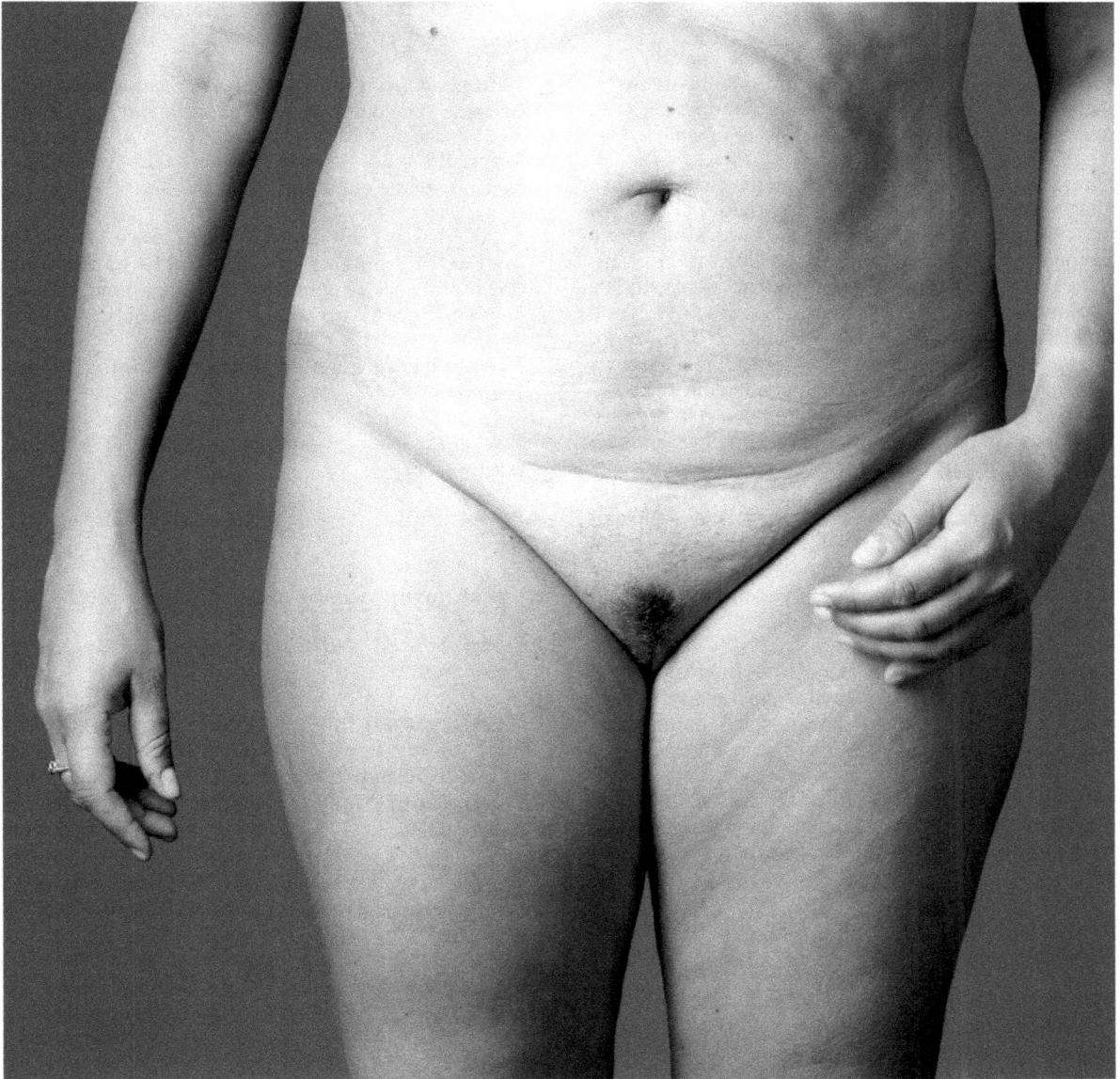

[T006]   The birth of my first child (section):

Induced labour: Approx. 6 hours. Head circumference 35 cm, height 54 cm, weight 3640 g, duration of pregnancy: 40 weeks +2 days. Totally different than expected, worse than feared.

Occupation: Seminar organiser.

When I hear the word "Caesarean section" the following words come to mind spontaneously: Risky surgery, missing out on the experience of birth, unintended, life-saving, once and never again.

Caesarean sections did not matter to me before the delivery: Because I totally disapprove of this way of delivery. Whenever I was asked, if I was afraid of the upcoming birth, my answer always used to be: "Anything but a Caesarean section!" I did not deal with this alternative way of delivery because it was out of the question as far as I was concerned. But deep inside me the Caesarean was a topic after having a dream a few days before delivery, which made it plain what was going to happen. Although I do not believe in dreams, forecasting, destiny or anything like that, I took it seriously: I am sitting in a pool of blood with an open abdomen next to the bathtub in the bathroom, holding my baby in my arms – and I was happy. About a week later I am swiftly lifted out of the tub in the delivery room and placed, still wet, onto the operating table with no time to lose. Only the happiness took a little longer in coming...

The indication for my section: Undernourishment of the child. According to the "mother-child pass": "failure to thrive, high stage longitudinal position, pathological CTG, missing amniotic fluid, many infarcts".

Complications during the Caesarean: Operation needle broke, part of it disappeared in muscle tissue, found and removed after using an ultrasound scanner.

The very first eye-contact with my first child: During the operation.

The first intensive physical contact with my first child: Approx. 2 hours after the operation. I can't remember anything though! I missed the child in my tummy so much and could not get used to it being this baby boy lying next to me now.

I suffered from depression after the Caesarean: Because I could not really be happy about my child.

My child was injured through the Caesarean section: A little cut above the right ear.

I had health problems after or I have been having health problems since my Caesarean section: Could not walk without pain for a long time, am still numb in the area around the left pubic bone.

I would have preferred a natural (vaginal) birth: Yes.

I was afraid of pain during birth/of perineal trauma: No.

I was afraid of a possible Caesarean section: Yes.

I miss having a natural birth experience: Yes.

I experienced the Caesarean section as traumatic: Yes.

My Caesarean birth is seen as a fully-fledged birth by my family, friends and acquaintances: "It was a Caesarean" was a sufficient answer to "How was the birth?". The assumption obviously: Oh, unproblematic!

The birth of my second child (vaginal delivery): Finally something that I could perceive as childbirth.

My fundamental attitude on the topic "Caesarean": I am endlessly thankful because the Caesarean saved my life as well as my son's. As the only solution: perfect! For any other reason: totally unacceptable!

My Caesarean scar (length approx. 15 cm):

Sometimes I'm sure the scar must be noticeable under my bikini bottom because a bulge has developed on the left side. If that is the case – which I do not think – then I am proud of this scar. And of only having "used" it once.

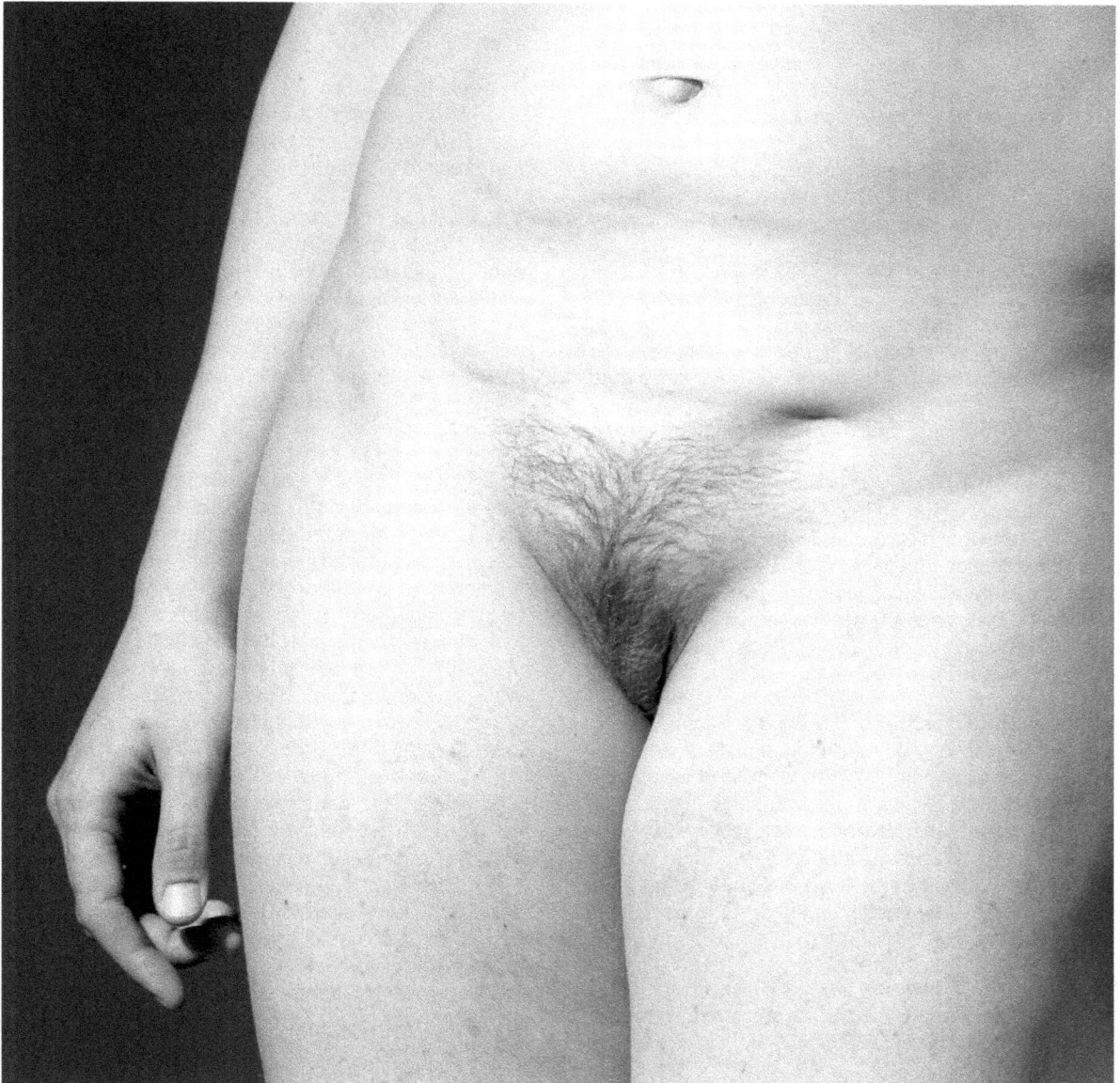

[T 145]   Now I know both:

Medically botched birth and natural birth. I am convinced, after the distress experienced with my first child, birth would be a lot less complicated if physicians did not interfere that much. Children come from women's strength!

Occupation: Physician.

When I hear the word "Caesarean section" the following words come to mind spontaneously: Mostly the result of too much interference by physicians, naked like a piece of meat strapped down with the legs apart, helpless, incapacitated, humiliated, humbled, extremely hurt, deprived of my womanliness, life-saving only in the minority of cases, for the majority unnecessary.

The birth of my first child (section): Induced labour: Approx. 20 hours. Head circumference 34 cm, height 50 cm, weight 3100 g, duration of pregnancy: 42 weeks corrected, 40 weeks +2 days calculated date. Readjustment! of the date of delivery – 12 days earlier – in the early stages of pregnancy by the gynaecologist! Exceeding the expected date of birth, the exact date of ovulation and conception were irrelevant to the physician. After hinting that I mistrust the altered term indicated by ultrasound, I was told off to the extent that I did not dare to say anything more as I did not want to be treated like a piece of dirt when giving birth. Induction, two days of waiting, induction repeated twice, 20 hours of horror contractions, epidural, Caesarean section: Traumatic!

Prior to the Caesarean I received drugs: Prostin gel and Propes-vag. pills for induction, Paspertum IV against excessive vomiting, Standacillin IV (antibiotic) against a raised temperature and feared increase in infection (physicians have not yet discovered that labour is heavy muscular work and warmth may occur), Syntocinon IV (for contractions) due to weak contractions, Tocolytics (contraction inhibitor) for contractions that are too strong, epidural.

I ascribe the following peculiarities of my child to the Caesarean birth: Restlessness, remarkable alertness, as if he could not trust the world, well, he was violently driven out of paradise, ultimately forcibly by knife.

A Caesarean birth has negative effects on the child: Because the natural way is always the better one, also gentler. And because the drugs which are pumped into the mother are not healthy for the child.

The birth of my second child (vaginal delivery): From the beginning I fought determinedly against bringing the term forward and against an induction; searched for my own midwife who came along to the hospital at our cost and it paid off! 13 days after my due date our daughter was happily delivered, totally naturally – without induction, without a drip, without painkillers. I would immediately have another child this way.

Additional notes: A good midwife is important and also the antenatal instruction, best with the same midwife and together with one's partner because that creates trust and makes it easy to let go when giving birth. Women have good intuition – unfortunately it is often overlaid with fears stoked by physicians, the woman is alienated and completely helpless. The medical fraternity way too often likes to present itself as a lifesaver. With my second child I fought from the beginning, insisted on my due date because they wanted to bring it forward again and had to put up with them calling me stubborn at the "mother-child pass examination". My child made the most of the pregnancy right up to the last day. I refused the induction on the 12th day beyond term and on the 13th day the birth was a wonderfully natural experience. The child showed no adverse signs of being overdue and also the placenta was not calcified. Women, do not let anybody put you off, find allies, an available midwife, do not let anybody scare you! By the way: A well-planned home birth is just as safe as a birth in hospital, unfortunately not permitted after a Caesarean.

My Caesarean scar (length approx. 17.5 cm):

In the beginning I thought I would never want to go to a sauna or into a communal shower again. Yet, unless one stares intentionally, one does not see the scar. By way of the project of this book I approached my scar in a positive way for the very first time. That it can be photographed aesthetically, I find to be a totally new and interesting perspective.

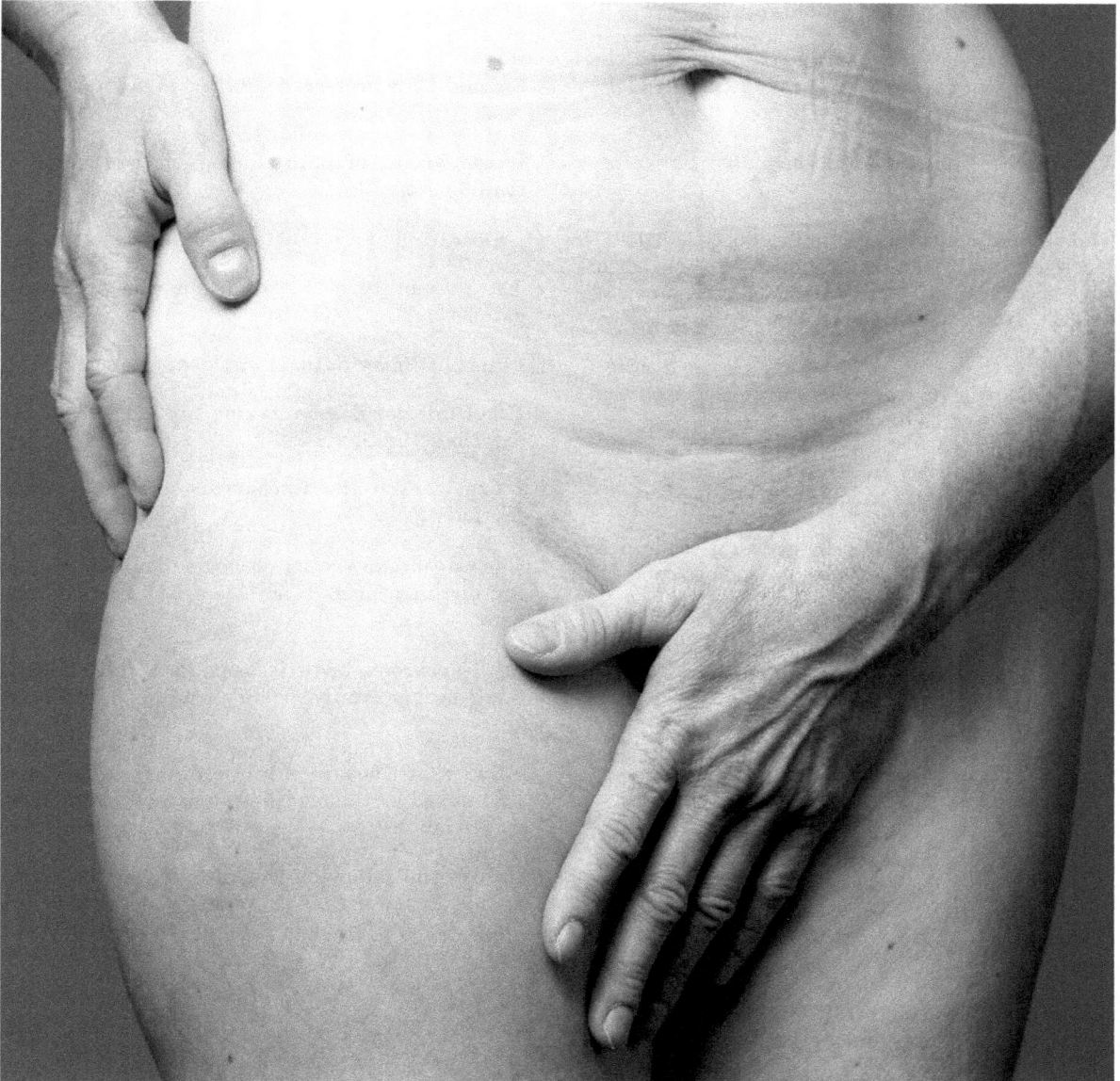

[T104]   I am glad:

That giving birth to my daughter worked out so well for both of us.

Occupation: Export Sales Executive.

When I hear the word "Caesarean section" the following words come to mind spontaneously: Lifesaving, healthy child, necessary procedure.

I dealt with Caesareans intensively prior to my first Caesarean birth: No.

The birth of my child (section): Induced labour: duration unknown. Head circumference 28.7 cm, height 42 cm, weight 1484 g, duration of pregnancy: 32 weeks. I did not notice a lot for I was under anaesthesia and woke up in intensive care.

The indication for my section: Hospitalised with pancreatitis after being on holiday.

Prior to the Caesarean, I received drugs: I was on drips etc. for a day due to acute pancreatitis.

The Caesarean proceeded without complications: I was under anaesthetic. My readings improved after the child was delivered.

I had problems breastfeeding after the Caesarean: Child was in hospital for 6 weeks – milk dried up. I did not breastfeed.

The very first eye-contact and intensive physical contact with my child: Approx. 48 hours after the operation.

I suffered from depression after the Caesarean: No.

The Caesarean interfered with the mother-child bonding: No.

My child had serious health problems / has serious health problems now: No

The Caesarean gives me the feeling of not having done everything for my child: No.

I would have preferred a natural (vaginal) birth: Yes.

I was afraid of pain during birth/of perineal trauma: No.

I was afraid of a possible Caesarean section: No.

The possibility of a Caesarean was prognosticated: No.

I miss having a natural birth experience: No.

I feel inferior due to having missed out on the experience of birth: No.

I experienced the Caesarean section as traumatic: No.

The Caesarean section was the ideal way of giving birth as far as I am concerned: I cannot compare.

My Caesarean birth is seen as a fully-fledged birth by my family, friends and acquaintances: Yes.

I find that Caesarean section is trivialised and minimised by the media (newspaper, magazines, television, …): No.

Due to the following the rate of Caesareans is rising: Because a lot of women unfortunately are afraid of the pain during birth or have their children delivered earlier.

My Caesarean scar (length approx. 15 cm):

I feel it when the weather changes. My Caesarean scar did not heal problem-free because I have bad scarring. It is made so that it cannot be seen in normal situations. To me my scar is the sign of my daughter's birth. Because I did not have a choice I wear my scar with pride.

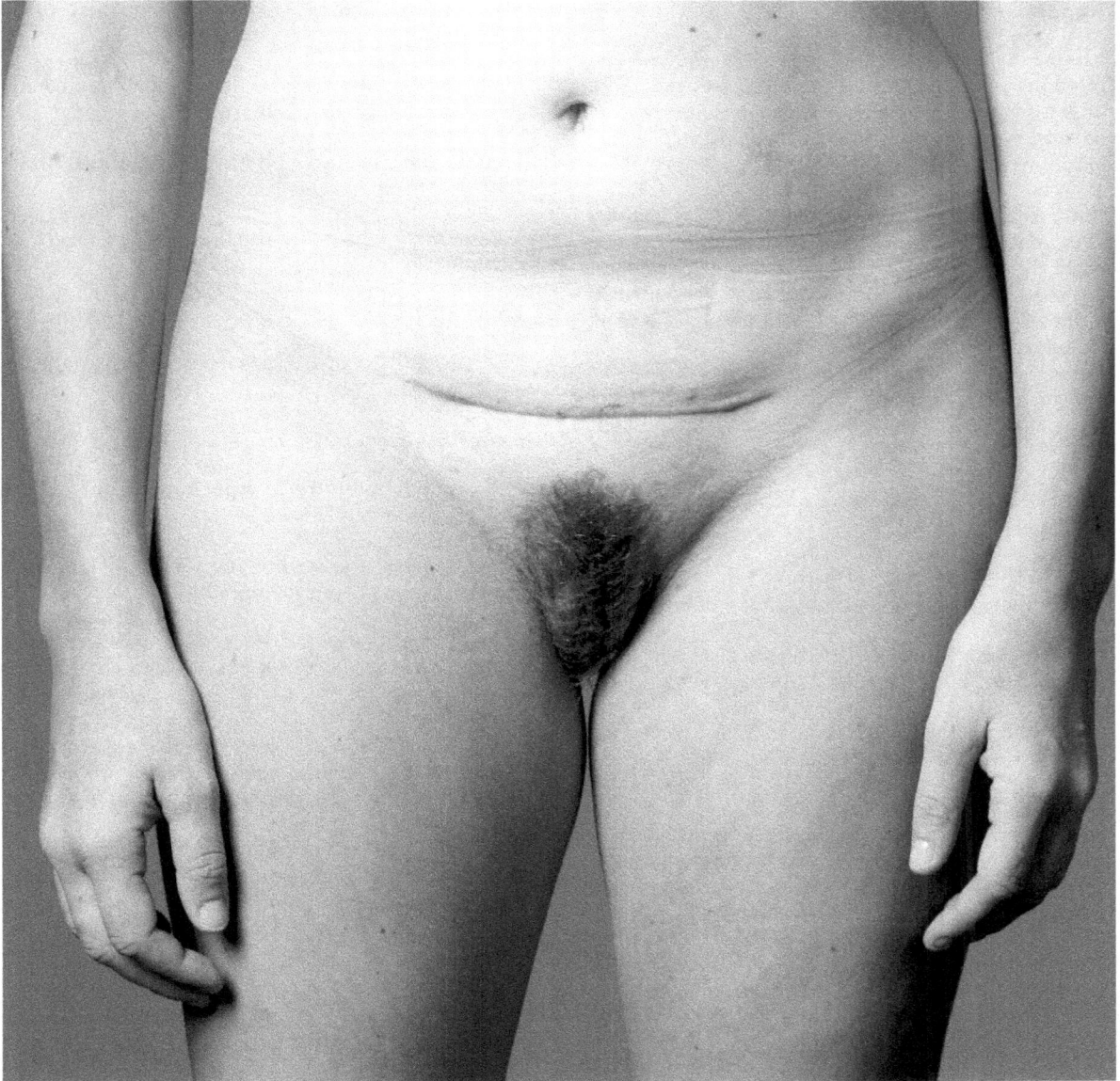

Caesarean mothers with one section

[T133] The Caesarean section was the ideal way of giving birth as far as I am concerned:

No.

Occupation: Employee.

When I hear the word "Caesarean section" the following words come to mind spontaneously: Surgical risk, no birth pain but wound pains, rescue, aid for survival of mother and/or child, missing experience of birth.

The birth of my child (section): Natural contractions: Approx. 6 hours. Head circumference 38 cm, height 52 cm, weight 3850 g, duration of pregnancy: 40 weeks +2 days. I pictured it differently, although do not have a problem with the Caesarean having been necessary.

The indication for my section: Cervix would not dilate, large head circumference, baby did not "slide" into the birth canal.

The decision for the Caesarean: Was made by me in the end.

Prior to the Caesarean, I received drugs: Antibiotics due to the premature rupture of membranes.

The first intensive physical contact with my child: Approx. 30 minutes after the operation.

I was able to breastfeed without difficulty after the Caesarean: I breastfed for more than six months.

The Caesarean interfered with the mother-child bonding: Due to the wound pains in the beginning it is not possible to care for your baby the way you would want to.

I suffered from depression after the Caesarean: No.

My child had health problems / has health problems now: No

I noticed peculiarities in my child, which I ascribe to the Caesarean birth: No.

I would have preferred a natural (vaginal) birth: Yes.

I was afraid of pain during birth/of perineal trauma: No.

I was afraid of a possible Caesarean section: No.

The possibility of a Caesarean was prognosticated: No.

I miss having a natural birth experience: No.

I feel inferior due to having missed out on the experience of birth: No.

The Caesarean gives me the feeling of not having done everything for my child: No.

A Caesarean section does not have negative effects on the child: But if possible the contractions should be awaited.

Due to the following the rate of Caesareans is rising: I am not able to relate to that. In my circle of acquaintances no one has ever had a Caesarean.

My fundamental attitude on the topic "Caesarean": Caesarean only when it is medically needed and the mother's or child's life is in danger.

My Caesarean scar (length approx. 13 cm):

The way a scar looks ☺ no specific characteristics.

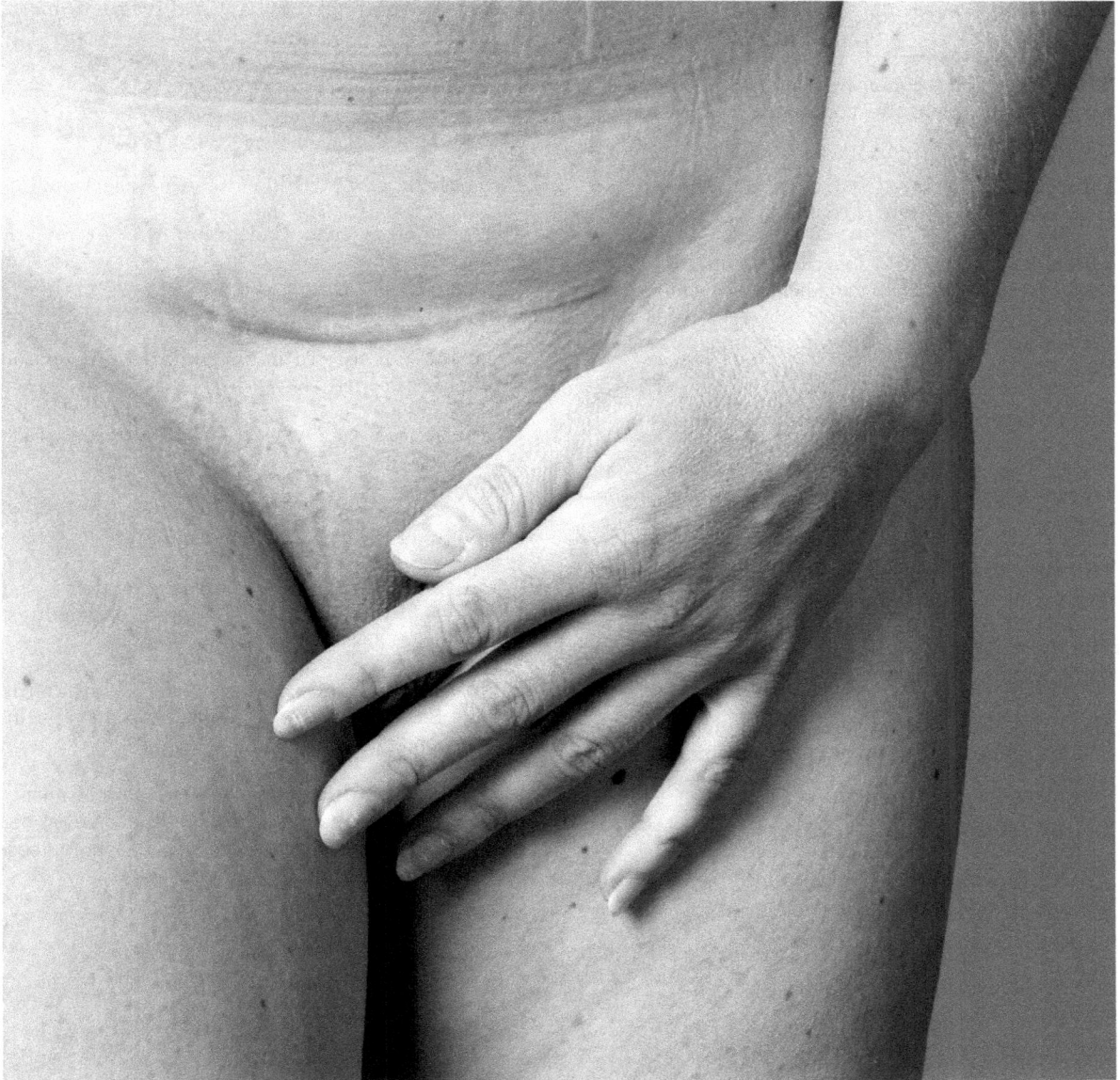

[T005]   The bonding took place with my husband:

I envy him for that.

Occupation: Consultant.

When I hear the word "Caesarean section" the following words come to mind spontaneously: Surgery, Julius Caesar, section without pain, lifesaving, epidural.

I dealt with Caesareans intensively prior to my first Caesarean birth: No.

The birth of my child (section): Contractions: No. Head circumference 36 cm, height 48 cm, weight 2250 g, duration of pregnancy: 38 weeks. Caesarean section due to placenta praevia and transverse lie of my child.

Prior to the Caesarean, I received drugs: No.

I was able to breastfeed without difficulty after the Caesarean: Yes, I breastfed for a couple of months.

The very first eye-contact with my child: During the operation.

The first intensive physical contact with my child: Approx. 25 minutes after the operation.

My child had serious health problems: Undernourishment caused by small placenta (small-for-date-baby).

My child has health problems now: No.

I noticed peculiarities in my child, which I ascribe to the Caesarean birth: No.

I would have preferred a natural (vaginal) birth: Yes.

I was afraid of pain during birth: No.

I was afraid of perineal trauma: Yes.

I was afraid of a possible Caesarean section: No.

The possibility of a Caesarean was prognosticated: Yes.

I miss having a natural birth experience: No.

I feel inferior due to having missed out on the experience of birth: No.

I experienced the Caesarean section as traumatic: No.

The Caesarean section was the ideal way of giving birth as far as I am concerned: Yes.

I find that Caesarean section is trivialised and minimised by the media (newspaper, magazines, television, ...): No.

Due to the following the rate of Caesareans is rising: Because women's self-determination is increasing and that is a good thing.

My fundamental attitude on the topic "Caesarean": Every woman should be able to decide on her own if she is in favour of or against a Caesarean section (as long as it is medically in order).

My Caesarean scar (length approx. 14 cm):

My Caesarean scar looks like a whimsical smile. It reminds me of being
a mom every day. It is easy for me to accept my Caesarean scar.

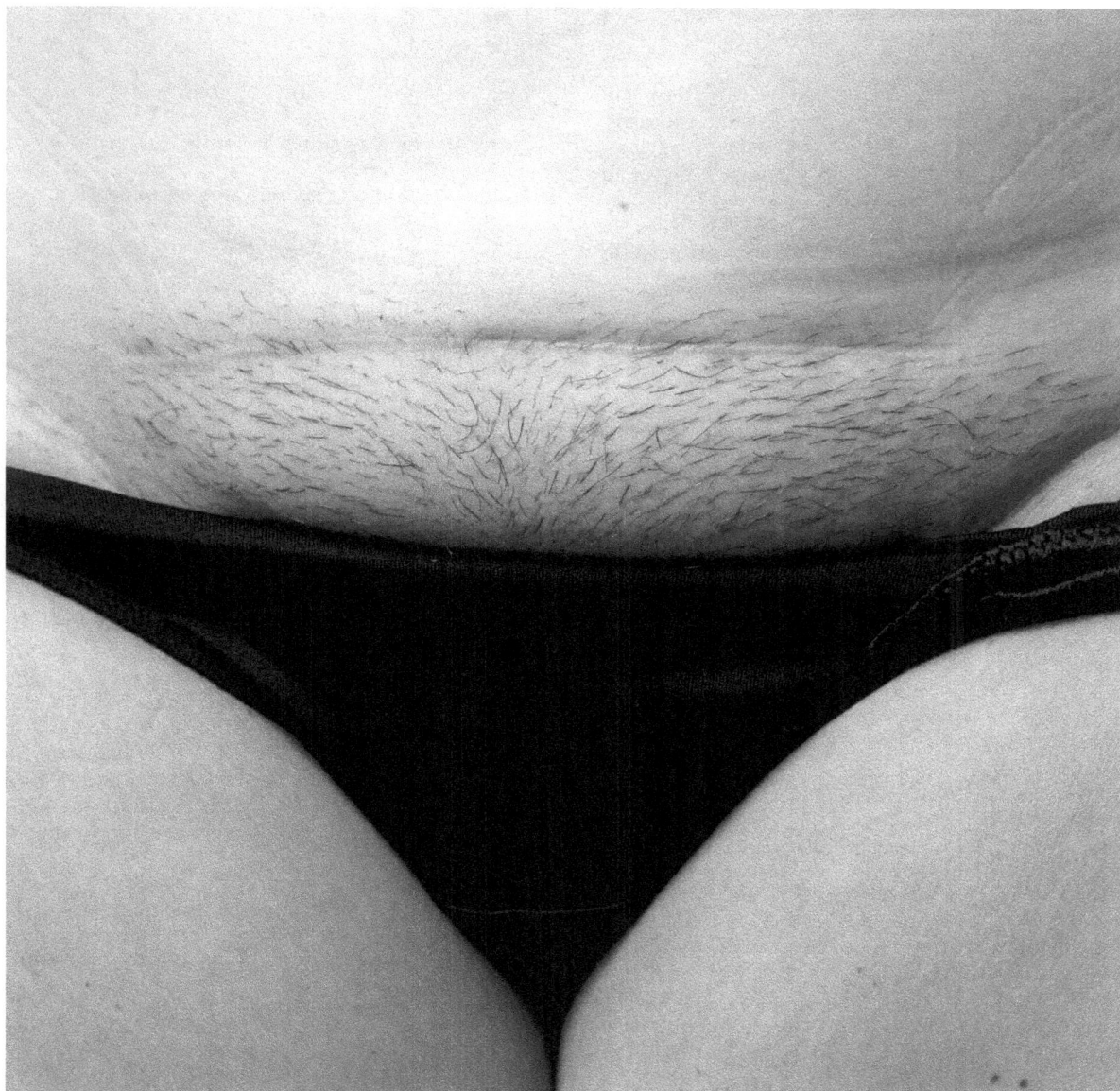

[T093] Intuitively I did not wish for a normal birth:

I was probably afraid of it.

Occupation: At the moment housewife, before distribution agent.

When I hear the word "Caesarean section" the following words come to mind spontaneously: Quick, efficient, clean birth, no contractions, no classical birth pain, scar, surgery with a long recovery, emergency.

I dealt with Caesareans intensively prior to my first Caesarean birth: No.

The birth of my child (section): Contractions: No. Head circumference: no entry in the "mother-child pass", height 49 cm, weight 3145 g, duration of pregnancy: 40 weeks. Very quick, without complications although there was a lot of agitation because of my illness (HELLP syndrome) in the first hours.

The indication for my section: HELLP syndrome.

The Caesarean proceeded without complications: Yes.

The very first eye-contact with my child: During the operation.

The first intensive physical contact with my child: Approx. 1 hour after the operation.

The Caesarean interfered with the mother-child bonding: No.

The Caesarean gives me the feeling of not having done everything for my child: No.

My child had serious health problems / has serious health problems now: No.

I noticed peculiarities in my child, which I ascribe to the Caesarean birth: No.

I was afraid of pain during birth: Yes.

I was afraid of perineal trauma: No.

I was afraid of a possible Caesarean section: No.

The possibility of a Caesarean was prognosticated: No.

I miss having a natural birth experience: No.

I feel inferior due to having missed out on the experience of birth: No.

I experienced the Caesarean section as traumatic: No.

The Caesarean section was the ideal way of giving birth as far as I am concerned: Yes.

My Caesarean birth is seen as a fully-fledged birth by my family, friends and acquaintances: Yes.

Society gives me the feeling of having failed: No.

Due to the following the rate of Caesareans is rising: Because it is quicker, cleaner, "less painful", partly easier to schedule, precautionary measure for mother and child also on the part of physicians, modern.

My fundamental attitude on the topic "Caesarean": Positive, with a further child I would request a Caesarean section even if it was not medically necessary.

My Caesarean scar (length approx. 12 cm):

A fine, straight line. Healed very well; just above the pubic hair, almost invisible. But a visible sign for my son, that he "lived" in mum's tummy and was taken out by the doctor.

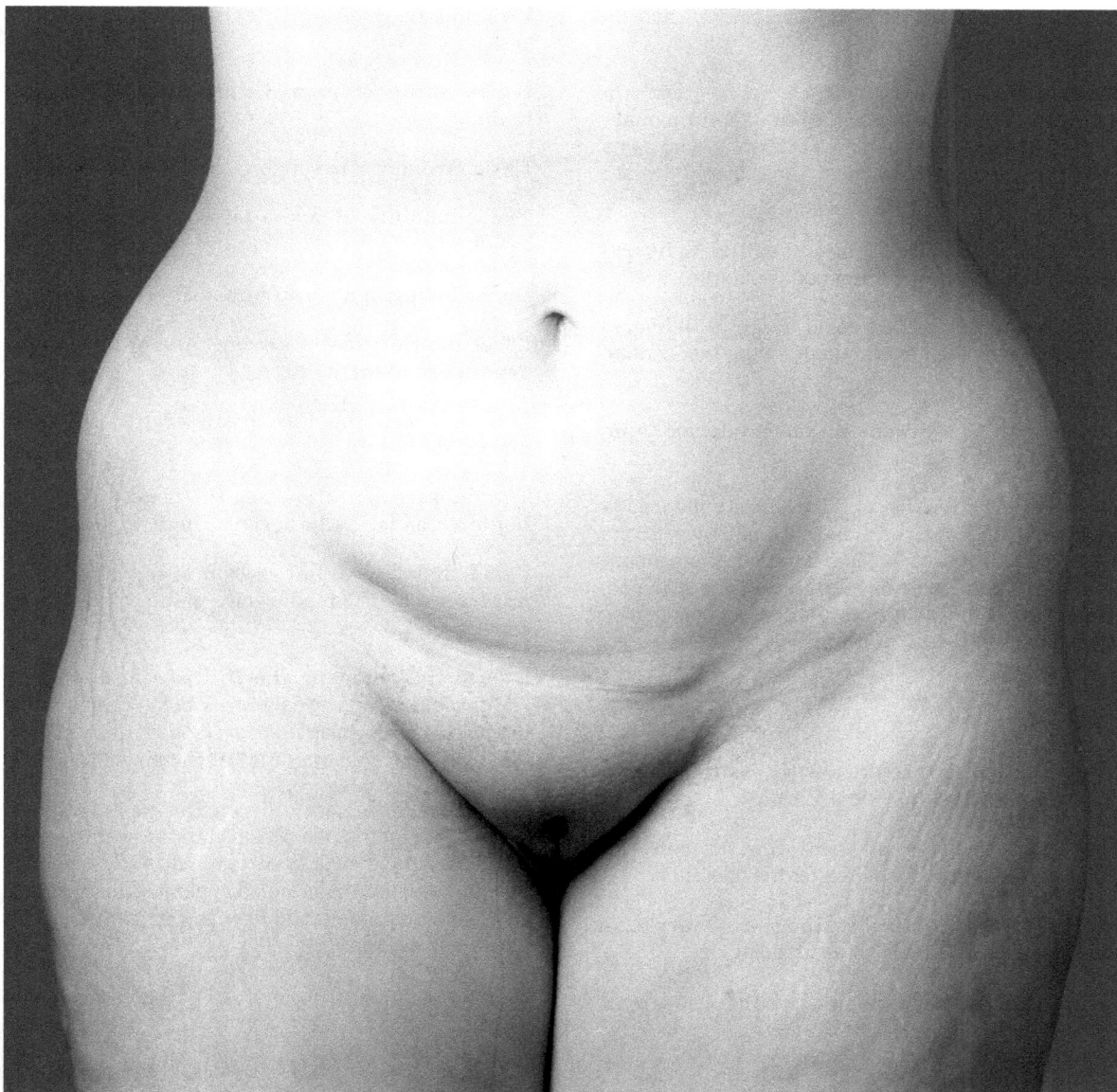

Caesarean mothers with one section

[T122] The birth of my third child (section):

I will always miss the strong, characteristic and very special first moment that you experience with your child after a vaginal delivery.

Occupation: Housewife & mother (before I had the children registered nurse).

When I hear the word "Caesarean section" the following words come to mind spontaneously: Surgery, missing the experience of birth, wound pains, when can I finally see my child "consciously"?, what a pity that it was "necessary".

The birth of my first child (vaginal delivery): Beautiful, uncomplicated experience of birth.

The birth of my second child (vaginal delivery): Very quick birth (within 2 hours from the first contraction).

I dealt with Caesareans intensively prior to my first Caesarean birth: No.

The birth of my third child (section): Induced labour: Approx. 30 minutes. Head circumference: 35 cm, height 50 cm, weight 3180 g, duration of pregnancy: 38 weeks. Intended Caesarean section due to a medical problem of the mother (atrium septum defect) diagnosed in the 34th week of pregnancy.

The Caesarean proceeded without complications: Yes.

The very first eye-contact with my third child: Approx. 1 hour after the operation.

The first intensive physical contact with my third child: Approx. 2 hours after the operation.

I was able to breastfeed without difficulty after the Caesarean: I am still breastfeeding.

I suffered from depression after the Caesarean: No.

I would have preferred a natural (vaginal) birth: Yes.

I was afraid of pain during birth/of perineal trauma: No.

I was afraid of a possible Caesarean section: No.

The possibility of a Caesarean was prognosticated: Yes.

I miss having a natural birth experience: Yes.

I feel inferior due to having missed out on the experience of birth: No.

I experienced the Caesarean section as traumatic: No.

The Caesarean section was the ideal way of giving birth as far as I am concerned: No.

I find that Caesarean section is trivialised and minimised by the media (newspaper, magazines, television, ...): Yes.

Due to the following the rate of Caesareans is rising: Fear of the vaginal birth. Women want to avoid the pain of birth which in my opinion is a very "important pain". The pain after the Caesarean is trivialised.

My fundamental attitude on the topic "Caesarean": It is great that the possibility of a Caesarean section exists in the case of certain indications although for me personally it is not comparable to a normal birth. I do not understand how anyone can request a Caesarean section.

My Caesarean scar (length approx. 15 cm):

I can feel my Caesarean scar. For the rest of my life it will remind me of this "different birth". Laser treatment was used on my scar in hospital.

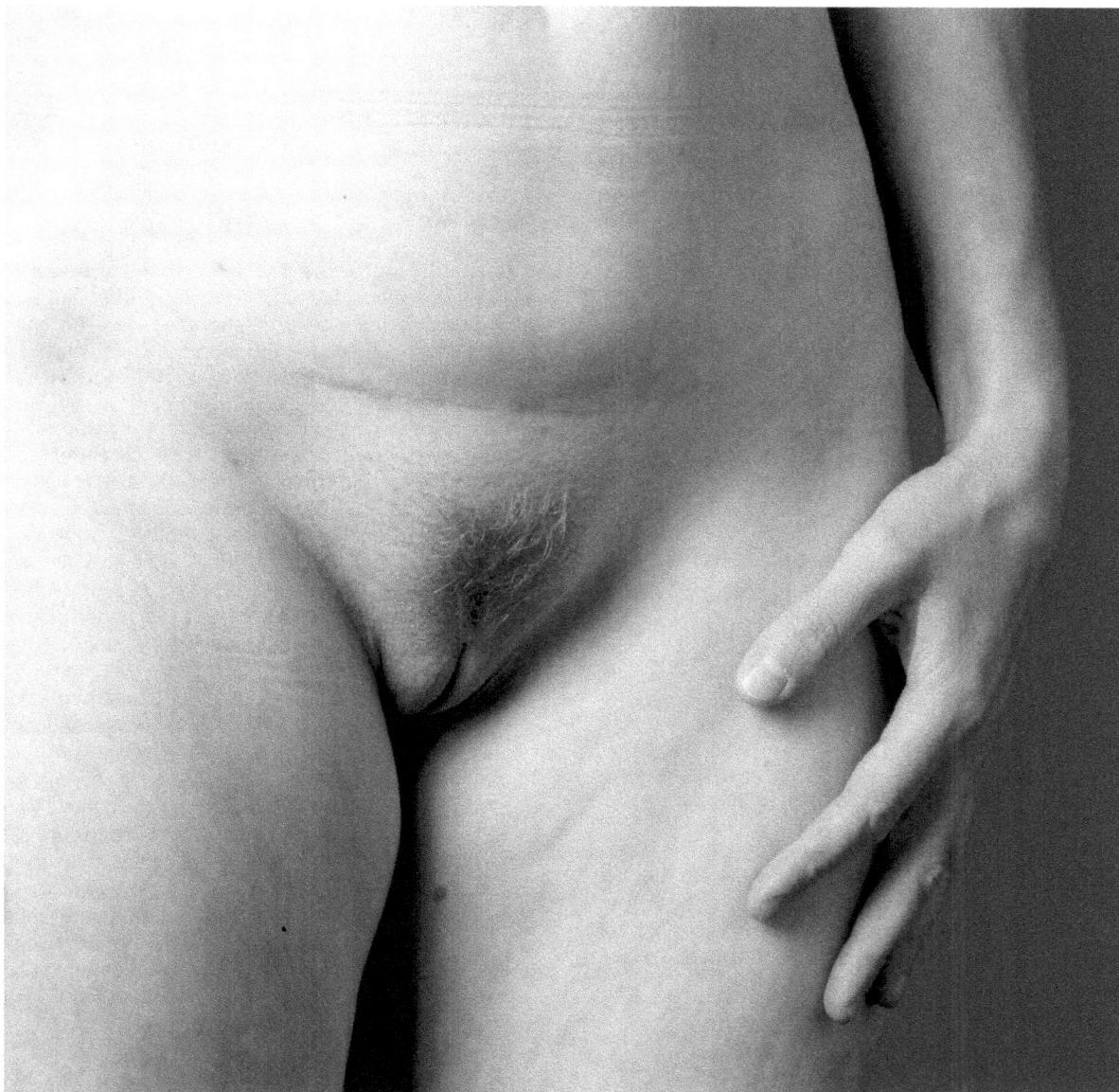

[T100]   My fundamental attitude on the topic "Caesarean":

Ambivalent for I do not want a further child to have to go through either my first, spontaneous birth (shoulder dystocia) or my Caesarean birth – although the Caesarean was possibly lifesaving for my second child. In my opinion the Caesarean should, anyway, only have the right to exist for use in such cases.

Occupation: Grammar/Vocational school teacher.

When I hear the word "Caesarean section" the following words come to mind spontaneously: Brutal, surgery, never again!, lifesaving, scar.

The birth of my first child (vaginal delivery): A nightmare – very rare shoulder dystocia (statistically 1 in 1000 births). 3 hours systolic phase of contraction. I thought my child was dead. As if by a miracle he was healthy and without subsequent damage.

The birth of my second child (section): Contractions: No. Head circumference 34 cm, height 51 cm, weight 3610 g, duration of pregnancy: 39 weeks +3 days. Due to the birth of my first child a Caesarean was recommended by different people. I was against it until one week before term – then I agreed. Section/birth proceeded without a problem but was traumatic for me.

The following people decided on the Caesarean in the end: Physicians, midwife, myself, my husband (father).

I was able to breastfeed without difficulty after the Caesarean: I breastfed for more than six months.

My second child was injured through the Caesarean section: Mark on the head (blue-red bruise).

I did not notice any peculiarities in my second child which I ascribe to the Caesarean section: Except for him being very clingy, wanting to be carried about extremely often and having a low frustration tolerance. (I do not necessarily ascribe this to the Caesarean section).

I had health problems after the Caesarean section: The blood circulation in my legs was disturbed; lochia congestion.

I would have preferred a natural (vaginal) birth: Yes.

I experienced the Caesarean section as traumatic: Yes.

Due to the following the rate of Caesareans is rising: Everybody wants to be able to rule, plan and control everything more and more– terrible in my opinion. Experienced both – the long wait (first child 14 days overdue) and the prearranging...

Additional notes: I am very glad that the possibility of the C-section exists and that the life of mother and child can, thereby, be saved. The method has become very advanced – all of this is very commendable. Despite this, I experienced the Caesarean section as very "brutal" – for me and my child. The child is literally "yanked out". In my case I was additionally reminded of my first birth – in a three hour systolic phase of contraction the child was literally pushed and yanked out – it almost did not survive. I thought that my second child would be born a little more "gently" by Caesarean – but it was also pushed and yanked out. The subsequent phase of follow-up treatment which took forever – until suture – was the worst. The child was with me for less than five minutes – I could hardly touch him. I was feeling terrible, I had problems breathing and with my circulation, the trivial conversation with the anaesthetists distracted me wonderfully but – did I want that? The "coffee shop chatter" of the operating physicians signalised that it was a routine procedure and everything was OK but the birth of a child is something so emotional, so special – I had to cry because of such insensitive superficiality.....

My Caesarean scar (length approx. 12 cm):

When touching my Caesarean scar I have an unpleasant almost painful feeling. When pressure is applied I feel intense pain. My scar is probably one of the smallest and most beautifully healed. Despite this, it bothers me – not for reasons of beauty but because of the way it feels. It all (the area surrounding the scar) feels very strange and vulnerable. It took forever till the shaved hair grew again (more than a year).

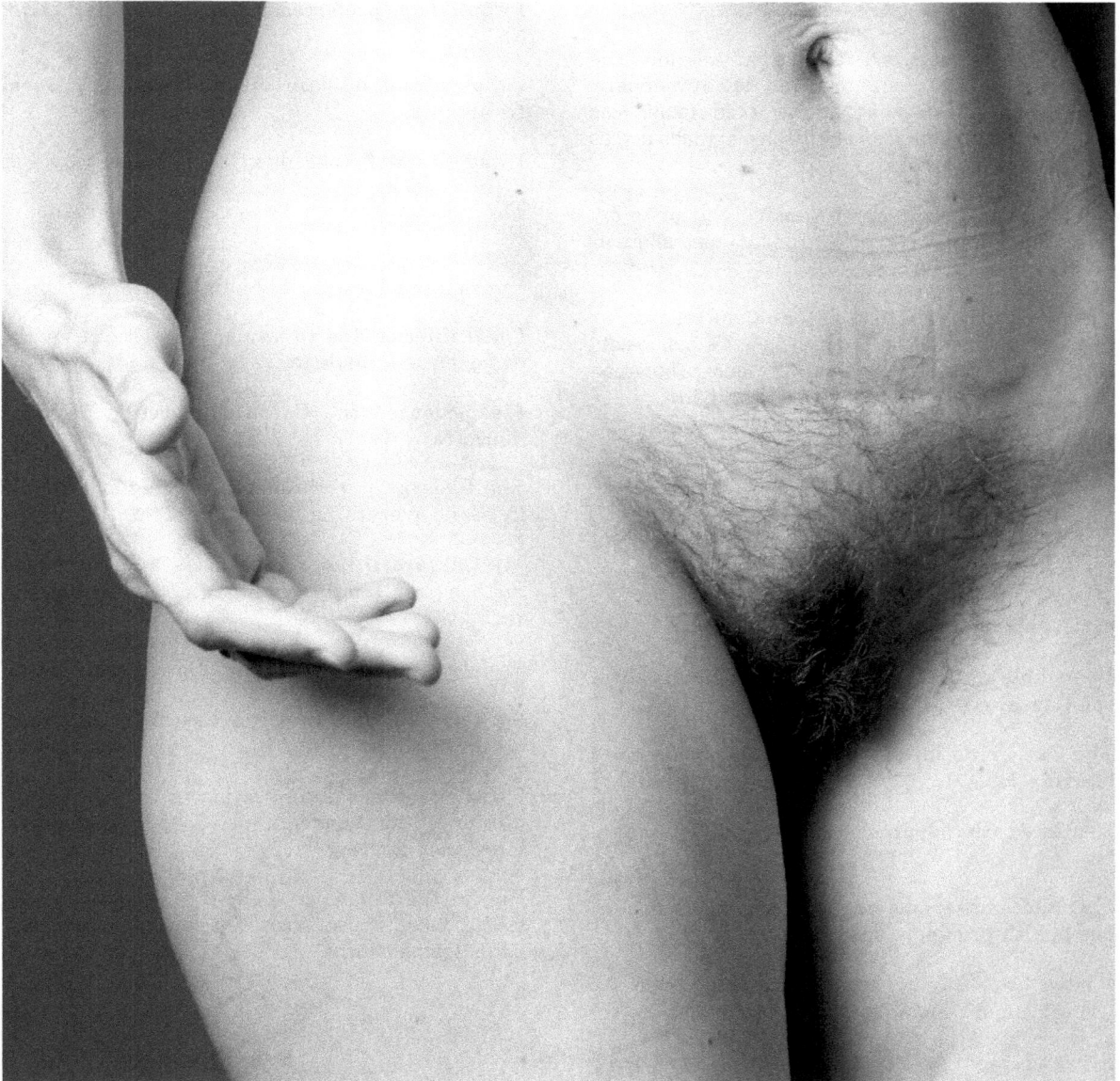

[T018]   The Caesarean section just "happened" in my case:

And was the ideal way of giving birth as far as I am concerned.

Occupation: Real estate agent.

When I hear the word "Caesarean section" the following words come to mind spontaneously: Safety, easy to schedule, mostly predictable, less stressful than spontaneous birth, pain spreads across a couple of days/weeks.

I dealt with Caesareans intensively prior to my first Caesarean birth: I like to be informed about all eventualities in good time.

The birth of my child (section): Contractions: No. Head circumference 34.5 cm, height 49 cm, weight 3320 g, duration of pregnancy: 38 weeks. The greatest gift on earth: giving birth to a healthy baby!

The indication for my section: Pelvimetry. Potentially problematic delivery.

The very first eye-contact with my child: During the operation.

The first intensive physical contact with my child: Approx. 30 minutes after the operation.

I was able to breastfeed without difficulty after the Caesarean: I am still breastfeeding.

The Caesarean interfered with the mother-child bonding: No.

I suffered from depression after the Caesarean: No.

My child had serious health problems / has serious health problems now: No.

I have been having health problems since my Caesarean section: No:

I would have preferred a natural (vaginal) birth: No.

I was afraid of pain during birth/of perineal trauma: Yes.

I was afraid of a possible Caesarean section: No.

The possibility of a Caesarean was prognosticated: Yes.

I miss having a natural birth experience: No.

I feel inferior due to having missed out on the experience of birth: No.

I experienced the Caesarean section as traumatic: No.

The Caesarean gives me the feeling of not having done everything for my child: No.

My Caesarean birth is seen as a fully-fledged birth by my family, friends and acquaintances: Yes.

Society gives me the feeling of having failed: No.

A Caesarean birth possibly has negative effects on the child: No.

I find that Caesarean section is trivialised and minimised by the media (newspaper, magazines, television, ...): Yes.

Due to the following the rate of Caesareans is rising: Safety aspect, trivialised presentation, "celeb" births seen as "ideal".

My Caesarean scar (length approx. 15 cm):

A smile. My child was born through this section/scar – what is supposed to be bad about that?! Since my delivery was only 10 months ago the scar is still a little red. Later it will not be recognisable anymore, it will look like a fold.

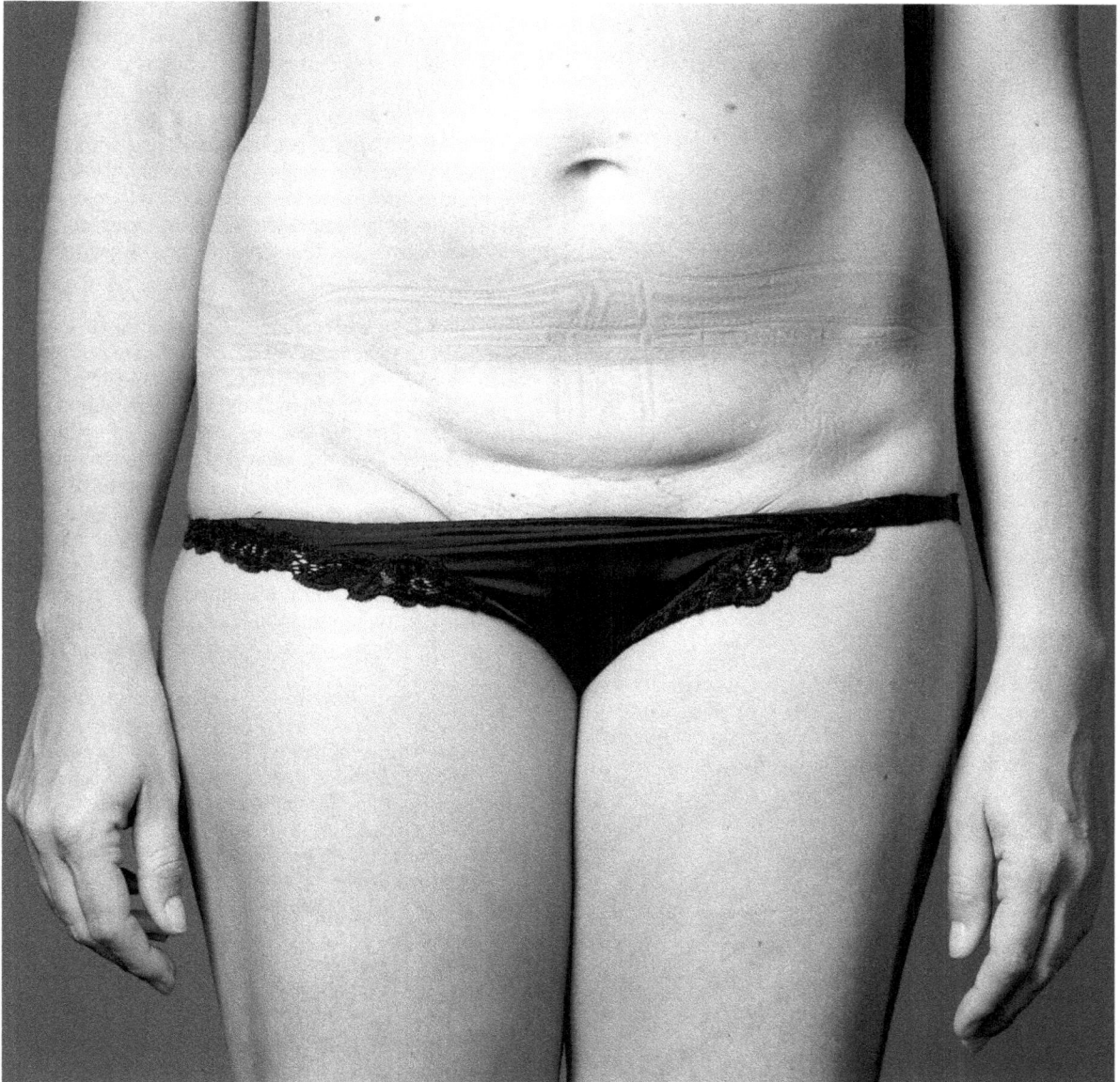

I pay for health insurance and am entitled to a quick "execution" of the birth without prolonged pain or effort. Medically doable things are done. In the case of overcautious medical indication or elective Caesarean section medical science is misused at the expense of a healthy mother-child relationship and a sound psychosocial development of the child.

Occupation: Registered physiotherapist.

When I hear the word "Caesarean section" the following words come to mind spontaneously: Injury of my body, farewell, wound pain, lifesaving procedure, blackout (due to anaesthetic).

The birth of my first child (vaginal delivery): Without complications, harmonious, in partnership, proud to have given birth relying on my own strength.

The birth of my second child (vaginal delivery): Severe pre-labour pain; disharmony with midwife; expulsion too quick; no complications.

I dealt with Caesareans intensively prior to my Caesarean birth: No.

The birth of my third child (twin, section): Natural contractions: Approx. 1 hour. Head circumference: 23 cm, height 32 cm, weight 714 g, duration of pregnancy: 27 weeks. Hospitalised in the labour ward because of preeclampsia; premature delivery; emergency Caesarean section due to placental abruption and intrauterine death of the second twin.

The birth of my fourth child (twin, section): Head circumference 22 cm, height 30 cm, weight 540 g. Death a couple of hours before the section despite examinations at close intervals (3-4 times daily).

The very first eye-contact with my third child: Approx. 12 hours after the operation.

The first (intensive) physical contact with my third child: Touching by hand on the second day (incubator). First "kangarooing" (child on my chest) on the 10th day.

I had problems breastfeeding after the Caesarean: Extreme engorgement in the beginning. Two weeks later – reduction of the amount of milk to almost nothing as I could only express milk at this stage and could not yet breastfeed my daughter due to the premature delivery. Previous experience with breastfeeding my first two children and personally studying literature, enabled me to increase my milk production once again. I started breastfeeding my daughter when she was discharged from the neonatal ward after 10 weeks.

The Caesarean interfered with the mother-child bonding: I, as well as my daughter, were "deprived" of three months of pregnancy. This time of bonding and comfort is lost. Birth should be a conscious experience of the first step towards mother-child separation where both realise the necessity and inevitability and consciously go through this process together and grow and mature through it. [...] Through the emergency Caesarean section the contact with my daughter [...] came to a, way too early, totally unprepared and violent end (at the same time it was lifesaving for both). The rebuilding of the mother-child bond took 10 weeks and was practically totally interrupted for 2 weeks.

I ascribe the following peculiarities of my third child to the Caesarean birth: My daughter suffered from anxiety and panicked when driving through tunnels by car (darkness interrupted by bright light = operation setting) in the first two years.

A Caesarean birth possibly has negative effects on the child: From a pre- and perinatal psychological point of view a baby, after a vaginal birth without complications, internalises a healthy pattern for handling all later changes as well as crisis situations. A Caesarean baby misses out on this.

I experienced the Caesarean section as traumatic: Yes.

My Caesarean scar (length approx. 15 cm):

My scar is emotionally very loaded. It symbolises the door to life and death at the same time. The pain of losing my daughter involved very severe physical pain around the wound when crying. The repeated opening and rinsing of the suture due to a haematoma meant "poking around in an open wound" literally and figuratively. At one stage, this resulted in a kind of shock related condition.

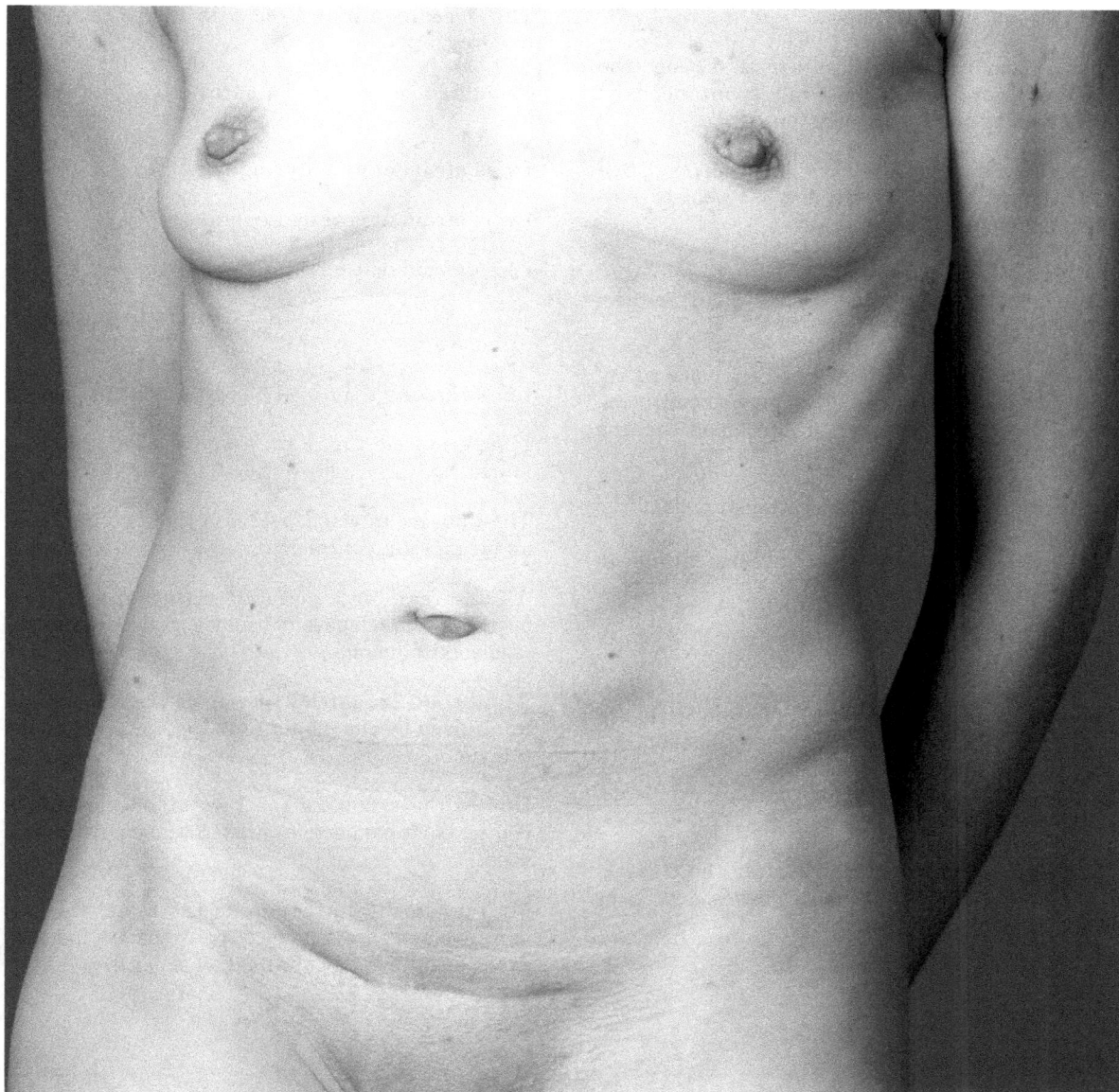

[T115] The indication for my section (third child):

Condition after traumatic births at the age of 22 and 27.

Occupation: Registered nurse.

When I hear the word "Caesarean section" the following words come to mind spontaneously: Safety, anxiety, pain, baby, physician.

The birth of my first child (vaginal delivery): Due to HELLP syndrome stillbirth in the 37th week of pregnancy, therefore very painful birth.

The birth of my second child (vaginal delivery): Very quick and almost painless birth, therefore mentally very strenuous.

I dealt with Caesareans intensively prior to my first Caesarean birth: Being an anaesthesia nurse myself I have been present at Caesarean sections many times.

The birth of my third child (section): Contractions: No. Head circumference n.s., height 49 cm, weight 3280 g, duration of pregnancy: 37 weeks +5 days. To me the most beautiful birth!

The very first eye-contact with my third child: During the operation.

The first intensive physical contact with my third child: Approx. 24 hours after the operation.

My third child has serious health problems: Adaptive difficulties.

I had problems breastfeeding after the Caesarean: Latching on and drinking problems due to my daughter having Down's syndrome.

The Caesarean interfered with the mother-child bonding: No.

I would have preferred a natural (vaginal) birth: No.

I was afraid of pain during birth: Yes.

I was afraid of perineal trauma: No.

I was afraid of a possible Caesarean section: No.

The possibility of a Caesarean was prognosticated: No.

I miss having a natural birth experience: No.

I experienced the Caesarean section as traumatic: No.

The Caesarean was the ideal way of giving birth as far as I am concerned: Yes.

A Caesarean birth possibly has negative effects on the child: Adaptive difficulties (body temperature regulation, breathing).

I find that Caesarean section is trivialised and minimised by the media (newspaper, magazines, television, …): No.

Due to the following the rate of Caesareans is rising: Older mothers, in-vitro fertilisation, safety reasons.

My fundamental attitude on the topic "Caesarean": Women should be able to take part in the decision-making regarding the method of delivery.

My Caesarean scar (length approx. 15 cm):

My Caesarean scar healed without a problem. I cannot feel my
Caesarean scar. My Caesarean scar is a very fine line, almost
invisible. It is easy for me to accept my Caesarean scar.

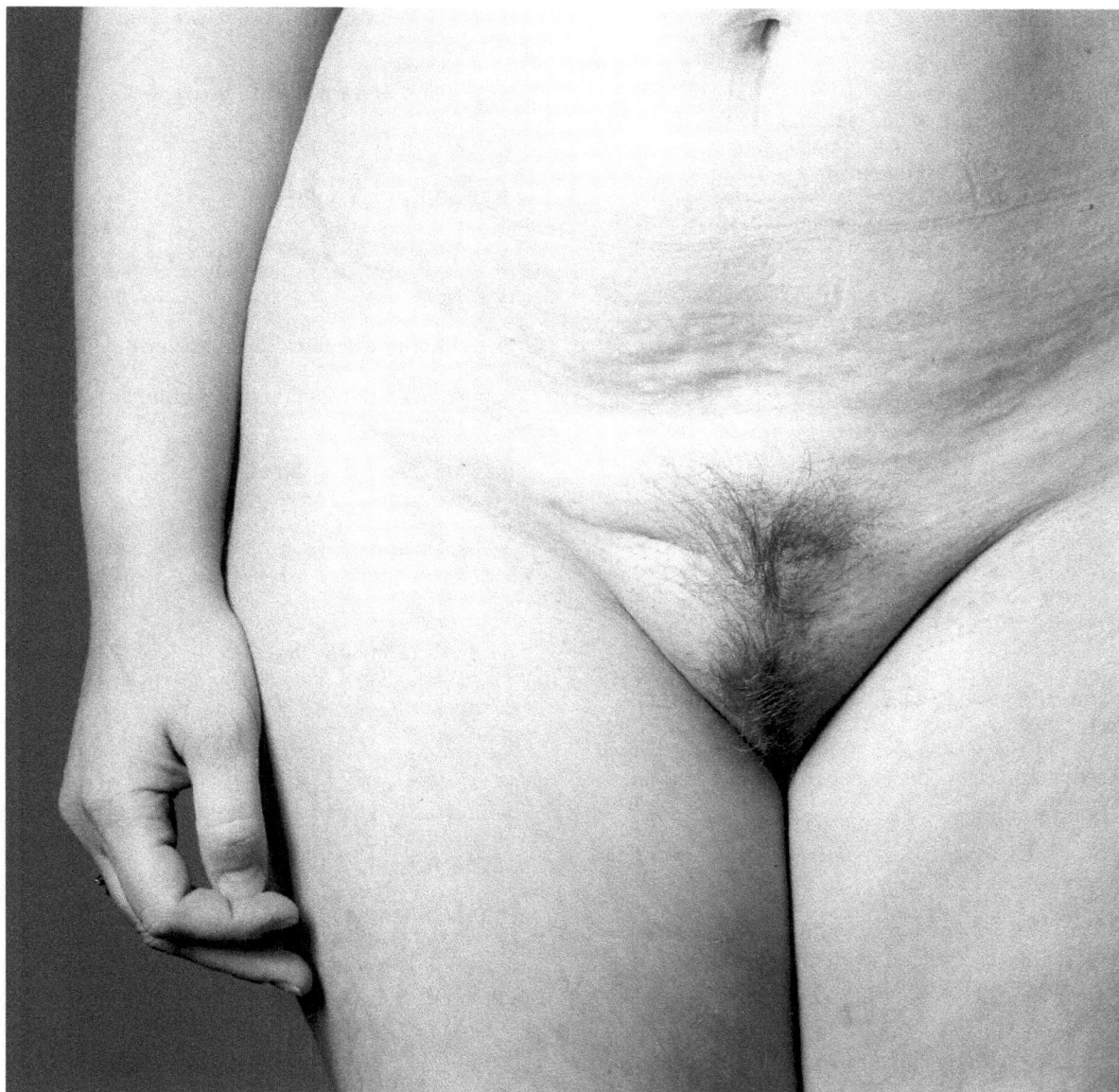

Caesarean mothers with one section

[T091] The Caesarean section did not significantly interfere with the mother-child bonding:

I myself did not find it disturbing – you can still cuddle the baby later.

Occupation: Master of rural home management.

When I hear the word "Caesarean section" the following words come to mind spontaneously: Fear, no movement in bed, sandbag, getting up for the first time and taking a few steps, getting nothing to drink as I could not breastfeed.

I dealt with Caesareans intensively prior to my first Caesarean birth: No.

The birth of my first child (section): Contractions: No. Head circumference 36 cm, height 55 cm, weight 3780 g, duration of pregnancy: 43 weeks. I was 17 years of age, was not prepared for a Caesarean section. The obstetricians in hospital wanted to wait with the delivery, until my general practitioner told them on the telephone that the term was correct. With my daughter the calculated term was the 16th of May – she was only born in the middle of June, almost a 10-month-baby. A physician told me that the amniotic fluid was purulent. They would have induced labour days before but I did not have any contractions. The cardiotocograph showed huge contractions but I did not feel any.

The indication for my section: The pelvis was too narrow therefore a vaginal delivery was not possible.

Prior to the Caesarean I received drugs: Labour was induced but nothing changed, I did not have contractions.

The Caesarean proceeded without complications: Yes.

The very first eye-contact and intensive physical contact with my first child: Approx. 3 to 4 hours after the operation.

I had problems breastfeeding after the Caesarean: I did not have enough milk.

I would have preferred a natural (vaginal) birth: Yes.

I was afraid of pain during birth: Yes.

I was afraid of perineal trauma: No.

I was afraid of a possible Caesarean section: Yes.

The possibility of a Caesarean was prognosticated: No.

I miss having a natural birth experience: No.

I experienced the Caesarean section as traumatic: Yes and no.

The Caesarean was the ideal way of giving birth as far as I am concerned: No.

My Caesarean birth is seen as a fully-fledged birth by my family, friends and acquaintances: Yes.

The birth of my second child (vaginal delivery): With my daughter I had a vaginal birth but was also in the delivery room for 30 hours as the cervix would not dilate.

Due to the following the rate of Caesareans is rising: Many want a painless birth. I think if you are well prepared you have a better attitude towards the Caesarean.

My fundamental attitude on the topic "Caesarean": I would only have a Caesarean done if there was no other way out. Although it also did not go so well with my second daughter I would, despite this, much prefer a vaginal birth as you are a lot more active after the delivery.

My Caesarean scar (length approx. 17 cm):

A nice straight section. The scar does not bother me.
I do not feel my Caesarean scar.

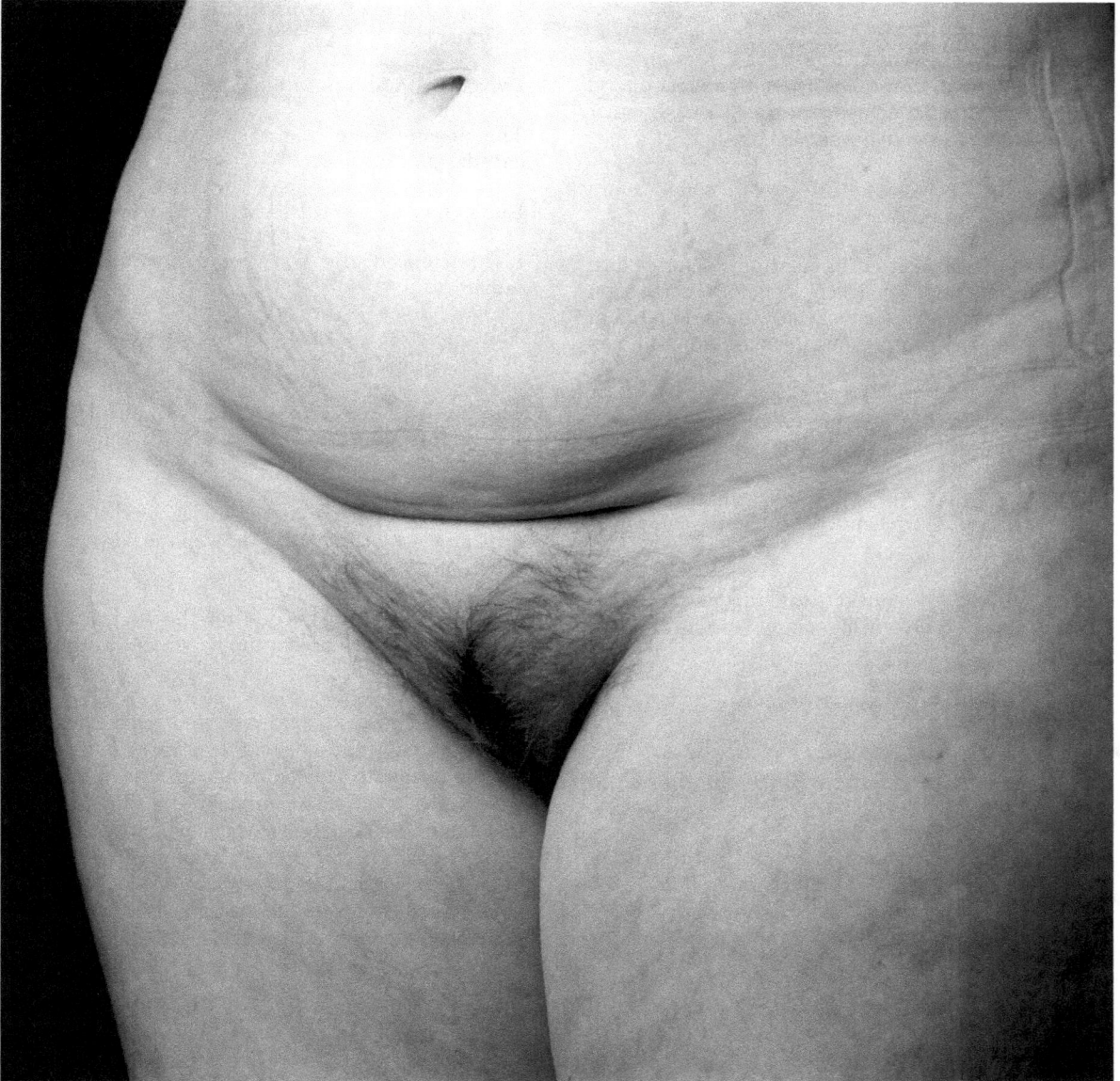

Due to the following the rate of Caesareans is rising:

Moneymaking + fashionable!

Occupation: Clerk.

When I hear the word "Caesarean section" the following words come to mind spontaneously: "Health" of the child comes first, fashionable, major invasive surgery, abdominal section, scar.

I dealt with Caesareans intensively prior to my first Caesarean birth: No.

The birth of my first child (section): Contractions: No. Head circumference 35 cm, height 50 cm, weight 3230 g, duration of pregnancy: 40 weeks. Rupture of membranes – no contractions despite drip. 19 hours of waiting, then section.

The indication for my section: No contractions, rupture of membranes; deflection; cephalopelvic disproportion.

The Caesarean proceeded without complications: Yes.

The very first eye-contact and intensive physical contact with my child: Approx. 6 hours after the operation.

I suffered from depression after the Caesarean: No.

The Caesarean interfered with the mother-child bonding: No.

I wanted to breastfeed after birth: No. I never breastfed.

My child had serious health problems / has serious health problems now: No.

I would have preferred a natural (vaginal) birth: Yes.

I was afraid of pain during birth/of perineal trauma: No.

I was afraid of a possible Caesarean section: No.

The possibility of a Caesarean was prognosticated: No.

I miss having a natural birth experience: No.

I experienced the Caesarean section as traumatic: No.

The Caesarean was the ideal way of giving birth as far as I am concerned: No.

The birth of my second child (vaginal delivery): Trouble-free. Contractions from about 7 p.m., birth at 2.35 a.m.

I find that Caesarean section is trivialised and minimised by the media (newspaper, magazines, television, ...): Yes.

My fundamental attitude on the topic "Caesarean": If it is necessary for the health of the child, yes to the Caesarean!

Additional notes: I had prepared for a Caesarean section with my second child. Two weeks before delivery the second child was "measured" by ultrasound. Weight and head circumference were within the normal range. The obstetrician was confident of a normal birth. Trust in the obstetrician paid off. After the birth of my second child the obstetrician explained the real possible reason for the Caesarean with my first child: psychologically caused, because separation (spatial) from the father of the child was scheduled four days after the birth.

My Caesarean scar (length approx. 14 cm):

"Bikini cut". Major surgery. The muscle was cut through.
Building up the abdominal muscles definitely a long process.
My Caesarean scar itches approx. two days before snowfall.

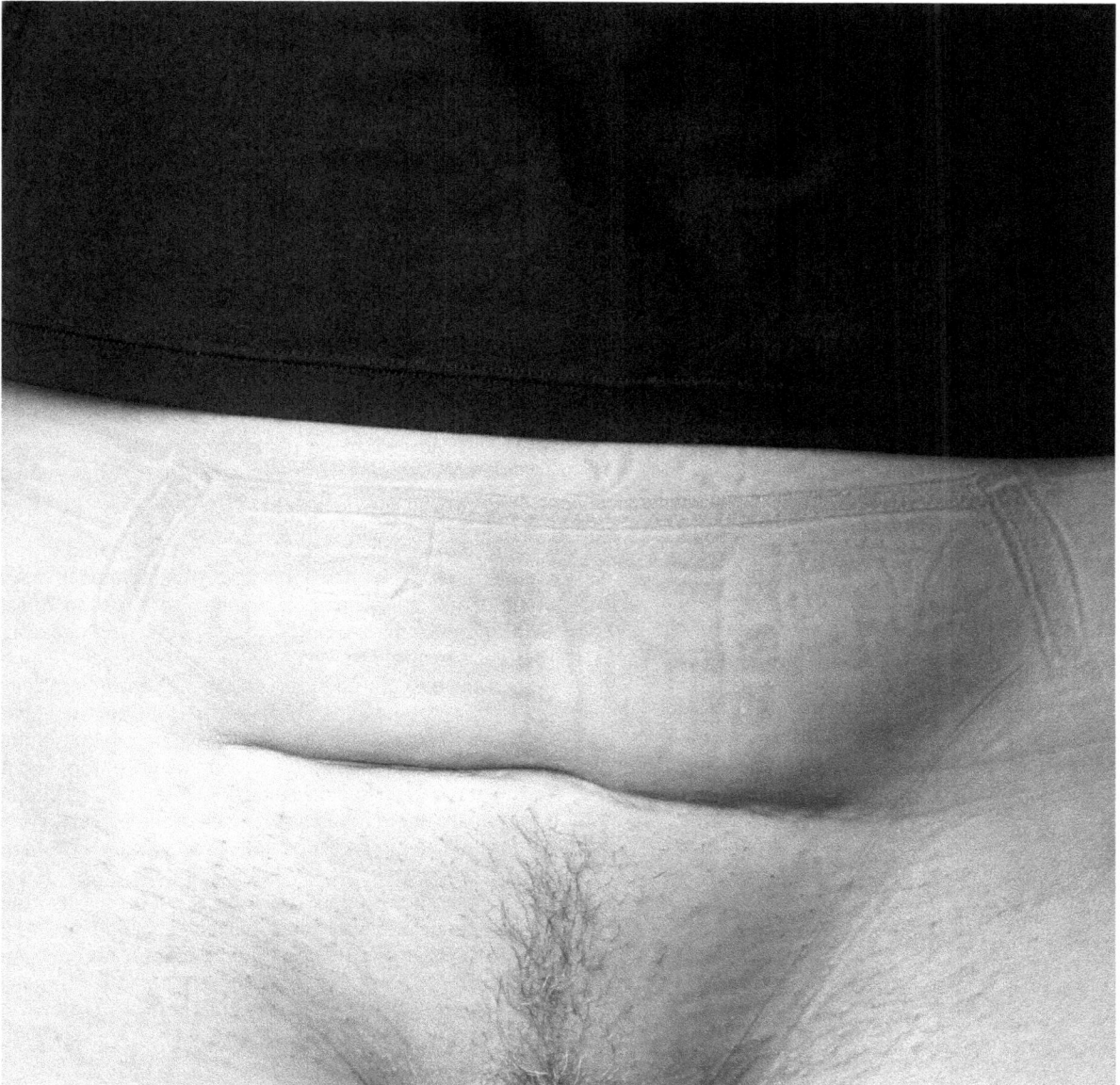

Caesarean mothers with one section

[T101]   When I hear the word "Caesarean section" the
following words come to my mind spontaneously:

Quick, What a pity!, surgery, anaesthesia, numbness, unnatural.

Occupation: Development politics instructor.

The Caesarean was not an issue for me: This possibility of giving birth was absolutely not mentioned in antenatal education, therefore came totally unprepared.

The birth of my child (section): Induced labour: Approx. 10 hours. Head circumference 34.5 cm, height 52 cm, weight 2844 g. 17 days beyond the calculated term labour was induced, did not work: Caesarean section.

The indication for my section: Failure to progress – cephalopelvic disproportion.

Prior to the Caesarean I received drugs: Homoeopathy.

The very first eye-contact and intensive physical contact with my child: Approx. 12 hours after the operation.

I was able to breastfeed without difficulty after the Caesarean: I breastfed for more than six months.

The Caesarean interfered with the mother-child bonding: Our son was carried around by midwives for the first 12 hours, by the father shortly after the section.

I ascribe the following peculiarities of my child to the Caesarean birth: A very restless baby who can only be calmed down by constant carrying. Maybe he misses not having bonded or he was yanked out of his "cave" too fast.

A Caesarean birth possibly has negative effects on the child: Too abrupt, disrupts natural procedures, anaesthetic prevents the first contact after birth.

I would have preferred a natural (vaginal) birth: Yes.

I was afraid of pain during birth/of perineal trauma: No.

My Caesarean birth is seen as a fully-fledged birth by my family, friends and acquaintances: Experiencing birth and general experience are missing, woman cannot join in the conversation.

Due to the following the rate of Caesareans is rising: The Caesarean is trivialised, "instant birth", women want to safeguard themselves against pain, physicians make money from Caesareans (?), the naturalness disappears.

My fundamental attitude on the topic "Caesarean": Good that it exists as a last resort, but should definitely be clarified as an "alternative".

Additional notes: As I was totally unprepared for my Caesarean, I insist that this topic be integrated in every antenatal class so that, should the situation arise, women do not feel so overburdened by the decision. I was too afraid to reject the induction advised by the midwife and the physician on the 17th day! (no miscalculation) beyond the calculated term. I am sure that this unnatural beginning and progression led to the Caesarean section. Would everything have worked out fine if I had insisted on waiting??? After the Caesarean I read up about it and saw photos of the surgery. I was horrified about the dimension of the operation. Women who do this voluntarily need to be made aware of the enormity of this operation. I regret not having had the experience of birth – I was so looking forward to it and felt strong enough for it. My only comfort was my son being healthy and that everything turned out quite well in the end – even though it would probably have been a lot better the normal way.

My Caesarean scar (length approx. 10 cm):

In the beginning I had the feeling the tissue was cut through, not penetrable, also concerning sensuality, eroticism. The harsh slash disturbed the otherwise softness of the abdomen/lap. I treated my Caesarean scar with "energetic" scar lotion. Approx. one year later I no longer felt it.

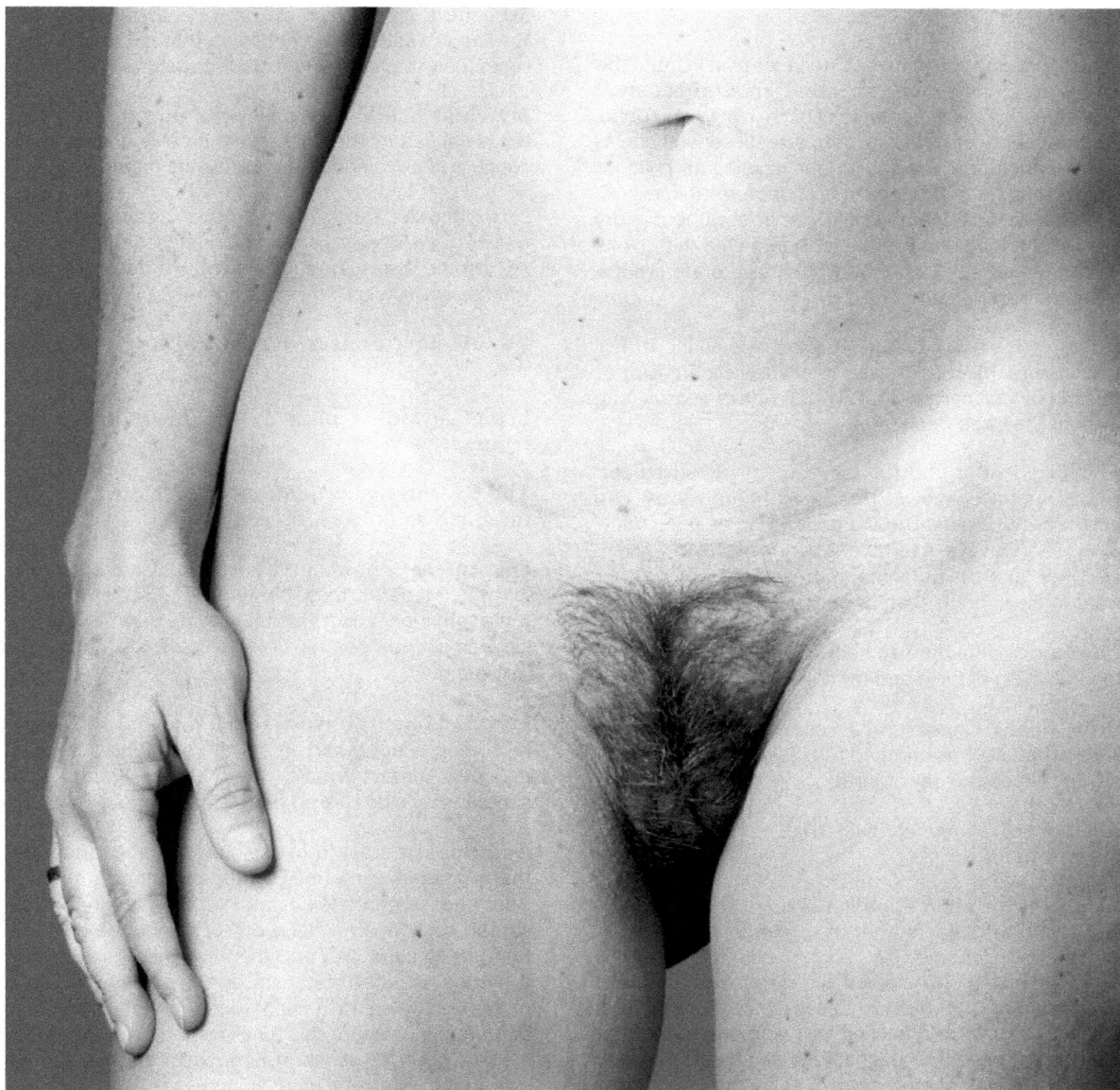

[T045]   I had health problems after my Caesarean section:

First the scar, I have had a hernia twice and my uterus also had to be taken out.

Occupation: Self-employed.

When I hear the word "Caesarean section" the following words come to mind spontaneously: I missed out on the experience of birth, I miss experiencing the beauty of birth, my baby's restlessness until a colour puncture at the age of four, missing my child for such a long time after the operation, a terrible experience for me, luck that my child was born without injury despite the long and terrible birth, am glad that it was there for "us" even though I would have preferred it a different way!

I dealt with Caesareans intensively prior to my Caesarean birth: No, was totally unprepared for it. But I know for certain that it would have gone wrong without the Caesarean.

The birth of my child (section): Induced labour: Yes, duration unknown. Head circumference 38 cm, height 53 cm, weight 4600 g, duration of pregnancy: 42 weeks +3 days. A terrible experience which I'd rather forget, just the outcome and my son I would never want to do without, seen as such – beautiful after all!

The indication for my section: The progression of the induction of birth and my condition.

Prior to the Caesarean I received drugs: Do not know what all. Was pumped full of ? from Sunday midday until Tuesday, day of birth.

The very first eye-contact with my child: During the operation.

The first intensive physical contact with my child: Approx. 9 hours after the operation.

The Caesarean interfered with the mother-child bonding: I was not allowed to see my child for the first 9 hours after birth, I missed this very much, the first eye-contact was not enough for me and created anxiety and worry inside of me.

My child had extraordinary health problems: He was so restless, did not sleep through once in four years, only improved with colour puncture.

My child has health problems now: I don't know if it is caused by the Caesarean, he often has a heavy cough and extreme fears of losing his mother.

I ascribe the following peculiarities of my child to the Caesarean birth: His restlessness, his anxiety, maybe also his eating habits. He does not really want to eat, it is as if he does not wish to live.

I would have preferred a natural (vaginal) birth: Yes.

I was afraid of pain during birth/of perineal trauma: No.

The Caesarean section was the ideal way of giving birth as far as I am concerned: No.

Due to the following the rate of Caesareans is rising: Modern times, being able to regulate everything with money. Not listening to your inner voice, physician's advice because of the money they get for the operation.

My fundamental attitude on the topic "Caesarean": If it is necessary in certain situations it should definitely remain a safe way of birth. Natural birth should always be ranked first.

Additional notes: In my opinion it is very important that women are informed as to how important it is to treat oneself and one's health with great care. A Caesarean section is an "incision" of the body which one first has to cope with and then live with. The scars of the body heal but the scars of the soul remain for a mother and also for a child. I know my child very well and am positive that this quick removal from the body created great anxieties in him, which he has not yet overcome. [...]

My Caesarean scar (length approx. 16 cm):

I just feel it very often, always have the feeling as if I have lost strength. The scar interrupts my flow of energy and has made it a weak point: 2 hernias. It always reminds me of this experience of unnatural birth. It hurts with weather changes, with effort and I feel it is a disturbing element in my body.

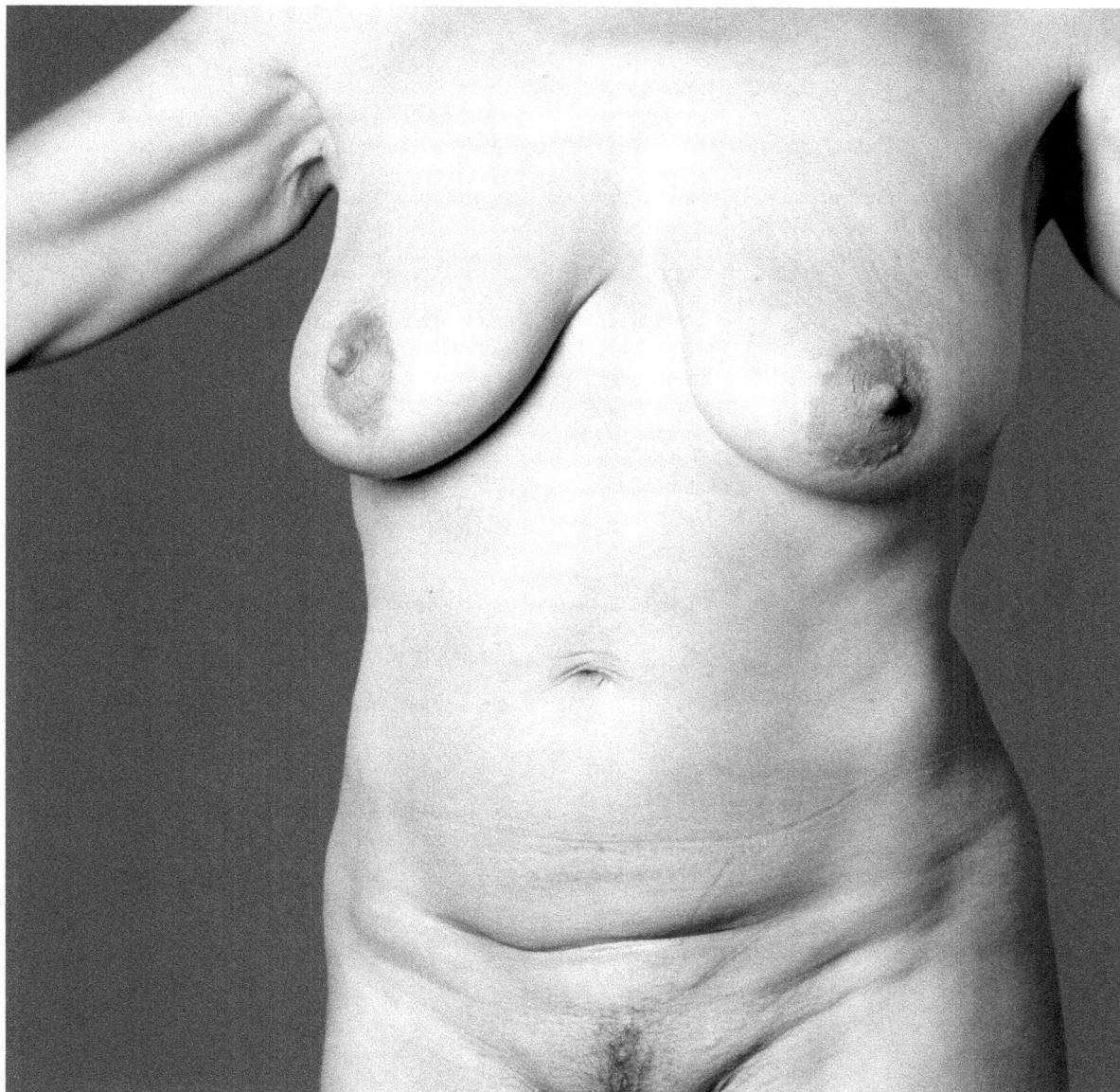

Caesarean mothers with one section

[T002] The indication for my section:

Acute infection of the bile duct and pancreatitis.

Occupation: Bookkeeper and payroll clerk.

When I hear the word "Caesarean section" the following words come to mind spontaneously: Feeling of guilt towards my child, good physicians, "bikini cut", scar, no breast milk.

I dealt with Caesareans intensively prior to my first Caesarean birth: No.

The birth of my child (section): Contractions: No. Height 44 cm, weight 2440 g, duration of pregnancy: 34 weeks. Due to premature labour in the 32nd week I received contraction inhibitors and drips. After spending two weeks in bed, inflammation of the gallbladder occurred. The following ultrasound examination showed that even the pancreas was inflamed. The physicians recommended a Caesarean section so that my child would not be endangered. The Caesarean was performed by emergency surgery, followed by removal of the gallbladder.

The very first eye-contact with my child: Approx. 3 days after the operation.

The first intensive physical contact with my child: Approx. 10 days after the operation.

I had problems breastfeeding after the Caesarean: I produced hardly any breast milk.

The Caesarean interfered with the mother-child bonding: My child was on artificial respiration for the first 3 days and spent another 7 days in an incubator. I could not cuddle my child.

I suffered from depression after the Caesarean: I felt I was a bad mother.

I ascribe the following peculiarities of my child to the Caesarean birth: Squinting caused by the artificial respiration. A colicky baby for 9 months.

I have been having health problems since my Caesarean section: Back pains, scar pains.

I would have preferred a natural (vaginal) birth: Yes.

I miss having a natural birth experience: Yes.

I was afraid of pain during birth/of perineal trauma: No.

I was afraid of a possible Caesarean section: No.

I experienced the Caesarean section as traumatic: Yes.

The Caesarean was the ideal way of giving birth as far as I am concerned: No.

My Caesarean birth is not seen as a fully-fledged birth by my family, friends and acquaintances: A natural birth is, by far, preferable to surgery.

A Caesarean birth possibly has negative effects on the child: A close mother-child relationship occurs with delay.

Due to the following the rate of Caesareans is rising: Medical fraternity's fear of failing.

My fundamental attitude on the topic "Caesarean": Only make use of a Caesarean if health and life of the child are endangered.

My Caesarean scar (length approx. 15 cm):

From time to time I feel a burning sensation. It took years before I accepted
it as part of my body. The long scar of the gallbladder operation is part
of it as the inflammation of the gallbladder triggered off the Caesarean!
Now I cannot imagine my body without these "signs" anymore.

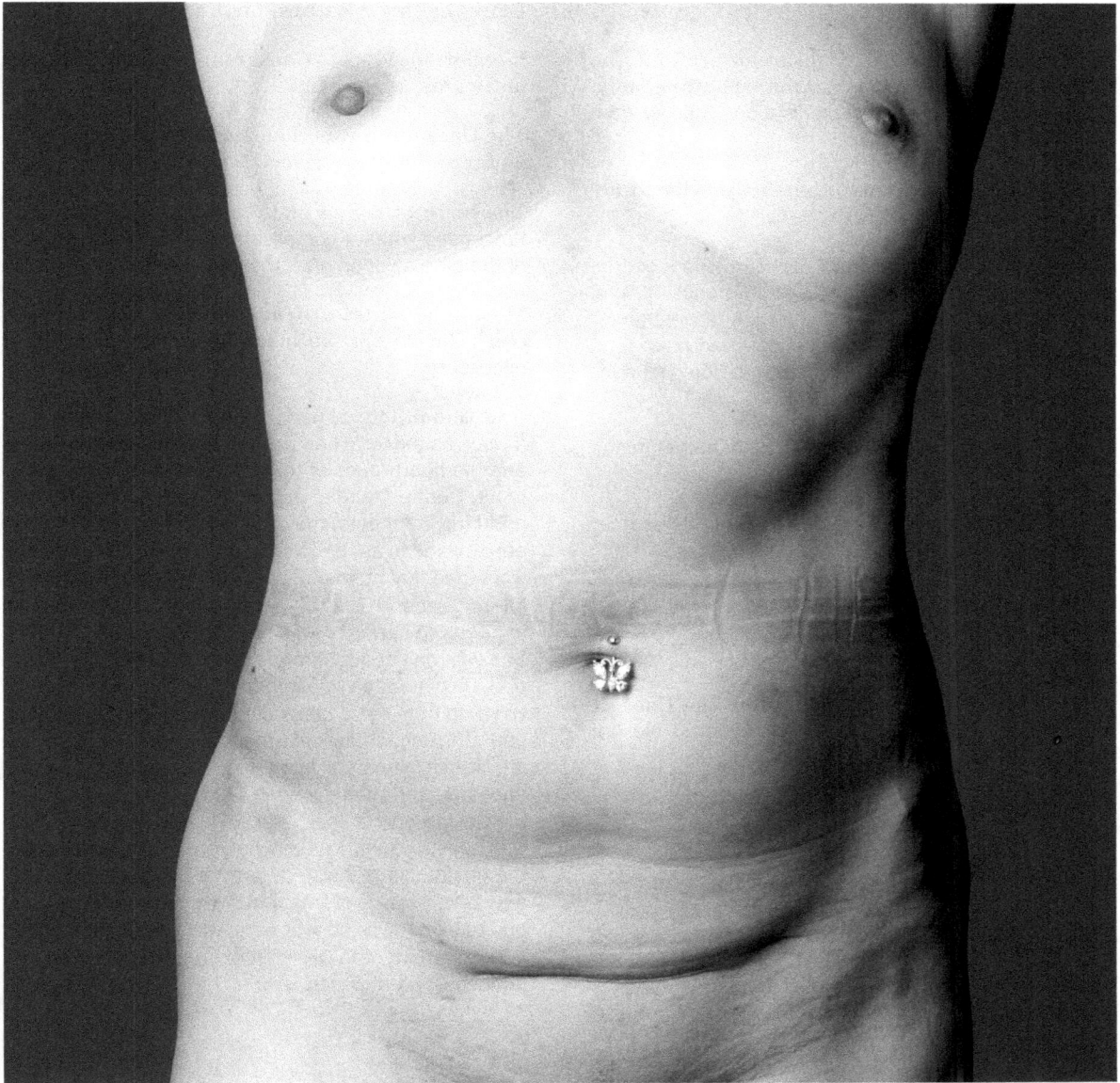

Due to the following the rate of Caesareans is rising:

The Caesarean is trivialised. This makes women believe it is the easier way.

Occupation: Travel agent.

When I hear the word "Caesarean section" the following words come to mind spontaneously: Complications, surgery, hospitalisation, child in danger, pain.

I dealt with Caesareans intensively prior to my first Caesarean birth: No.

The birth of my first child (section): Induced labour: Approx. 11 hours. Head circumference 32 cm, height 50 cm, weight 3440 g, duration of pregnancy: 42 weeks. During the third induction I had been on a drip for 11 hours enduring great pain before the decision to do a Caesarean was made.

The indication for my section: High stage longitudinal position.

The Caesarean proceeded without complications: Yes.

The very first eye-contact and intensive physical contact with my child: Approx. 14 hours after the operation.

I had problems breastfeeding after the Caesarean: Intake of antibiotics due to infection. I did not breastfeed.

I would have preferred a natural (vaginal) birth: Yes.

I was afraid of pain during birth: Yes.

I was afraid of a possible Caesarean section: Yes.

The possibility of a Caesarean was prognosticated: No.

I miss having a natural birth experience: Yes.

I experienced the Caesarean section as traumatic: Yes.

The Caesarean was the ideal way of giving birth as far as I am concerned: No.

The birth of my second child (vaginal delivery): Proceeded without complications. I was terribly afraid of the birth so soon after the Caesarean.

My fundamental attitude on the topic "Caesarean": Should only be made use of when medically necessary.

Additional notes: I had already been hospitalised for a week as the term had passed, I did not go into labour and the heart tones of the child were not in order anymore. During the third induction (11 hours on the drip enduring great pain) the decision in favour of a Caesarean was taken as the state of the child and mother had worsened. My husband, who was present, was not allowed to attend. But the worst part was that I woke up in intensive care and was not allowed to see my child. She was only brought to me 14 hours after the operation. Unfortunately you cannot object to this when you wake up from the anaesthesia. Three days later I got a bad infection, could not breastfeed and spent almost five weeks in hospital in total. In my opinion this experience affected the second pregnancy and birth, which took place only a year later. I was extremely afraid. I was again hospitalised as I had early contractions, but the obstetricians insisted that the child was too small and that it was a premature birth. In the end my second daughter was born at term with 2.64 kg and 48 cm and everything was OK. I felt extremely pressured and unnecessarily stressed.

My Caesarean scar (length approx. 14 cm):

My Caesarean scar healed without a problem, I do not feel it. It is easy for me to accept my Caesarean scar, I do not find it ugly.

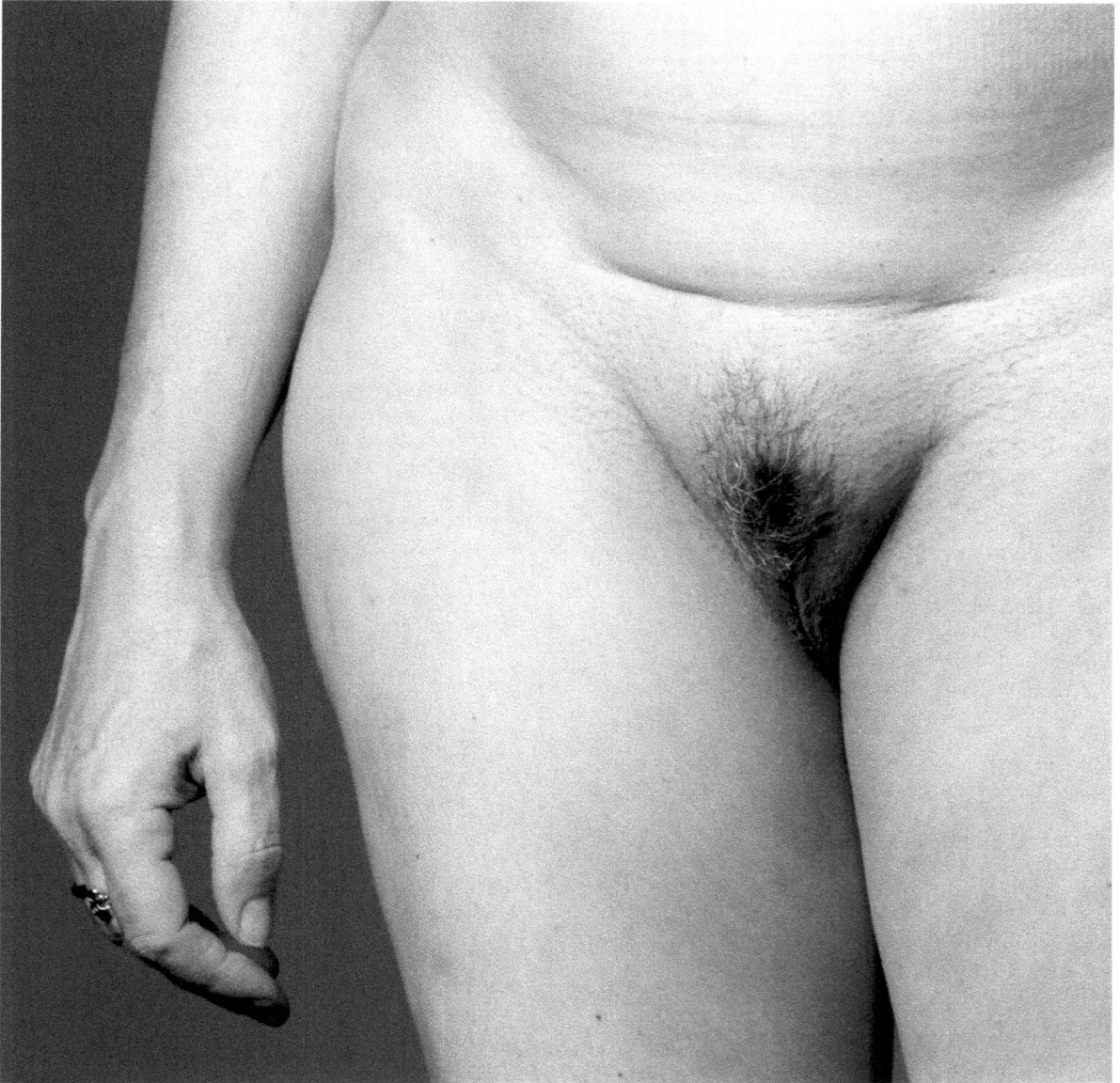

Caesarean mothers with one section

[T139] My wish:

Women should be treated with more dignity. I would like
to have my Caesarean scar operated on.

Occupation: Self-employed.

When I hear the word "Caesarean section" the following words come to mind spontaneously: Was a relief (normal birth in the operating theatre), was an exhibit (only realised later!), very badly sewn scar, scar totally disfigures abdomen, day after birth – ward physician apologises to me for the awful birth.

The birth of my first child (vaginal delivery): Was difficult, large head, physician helped with abdominal pressure, perineum torn and cut.

The birth of my second child (vaginal delivery): Pregnancy with a lot of complications, normal birth, perineum torn and cut.

I dealt with Caesareans intensively prior to my first Caesarean birth: No.

The birth of my twins (section): Natural contractions: Approx. 2 ½ to 3 hours. First twin: Head circumference 33 cm, height 51 cm, weight 2790 g. Second twin: Head circumference 33.5 cm, height 49 cm, weight 2580 g. Duration of pregnancy: 39 weeks. Should have been a normal birth in the operating theatre (!). After futile pushing contractions: Caesarean section.

The indication for my section: Occiput posterior presentation and transverse lie.

The decision for the Caesarean section was made by the following person in the end: Physician (professor)

The very first eye-contact and intensive physical contact with both my twins: In the morning during general breastfeeding time, approx. 7 to 8 hours after the operation.

I was able to breastfeed without difficulty after the Caesarean: 6 weeks fully, 6 months half the time.

I would have preferred a natural (vaginal) birth: Yes.

I was afraid of pain during birth/of perineal trauma: No.

I was afraid of a possible Caesarean section: No.

I miss having a natural birth experience: Yes and no.

I feel inferior due to having missed out on the experience of birth: No.

I experienced the Caesarean section as traumatic: No, just the incredibly large team in the operating theatre. Trying to have a natural birth in the operating theatre was not nice.

The Caesarean was the ideal way of giving birth as far as I am concerned: No.

Society gives me the feeling of having failed: No.

I had health problems after my Caesarean section: My eyesight weakened, this condition improved approx. five to seven years later.

Due to the following the rate of Caesareans is rising: Date can be easily planned for both parties. Possibly not wanting to experience pain during birth and the cost allocation on the part of the clinic!

My fundamental attitude on the topic "Caesarean": As in the old days: super when necessary!

My Caesarean scar (length approx. 20 cm):

It does not feel good and looks dreadful. It is badly sewn and attached to the intestine (?). The bottom part of my scar did not heal trouble-free. I suppose an inexperienced surgeon sewed it. In retrospect I think students were also present. There were so many people there. They did not inform me about this.

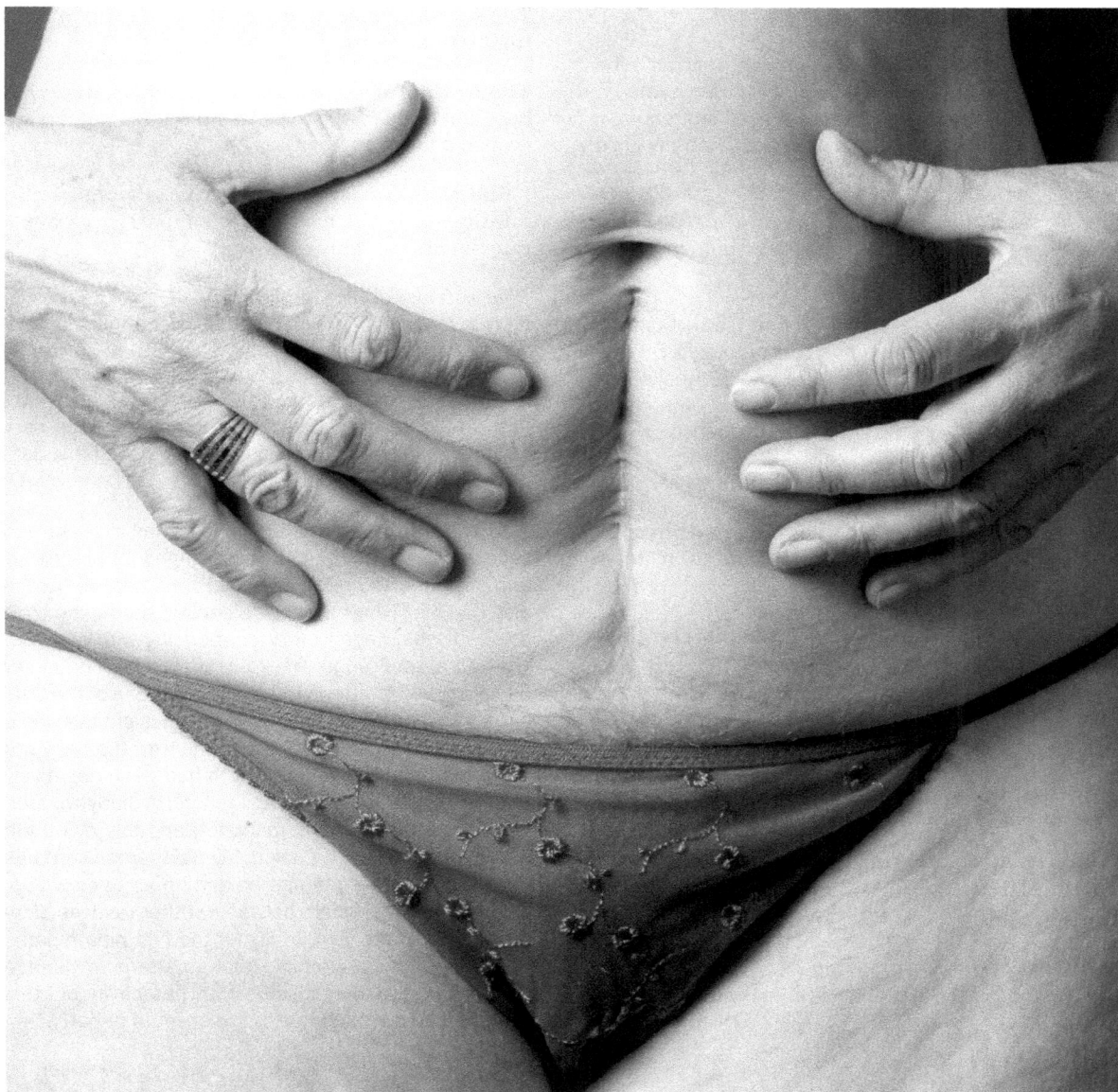

Caesarean mothers with one section

[T030] I dealt with Caesareans intensively prior to my
        Caesarean birth:

As I was informed by the physician prior to the birth, I read
a lot of information about Caesarean births.

Occupation: Dental hygienist, artist.

When I hear the word "Caesarean section" the following words come to mind spontaneously: Actually did not want it, hopefully it goes fast enough, no effort for my child, I am not awake when my child comes, many people scared me.

The birth of my first child (vaginal delivery): A trouble-free birth – the midwife was an unfriendly person.

The birth of my second child (section): Contractions: No. Head circumference 37 cm, height 53 cm, weight 3500 g, duration of pregnancy: 38 weeks. Unfortunately I could not reconstruct the day of the birth because of the after-effect of the anaesthetic!

The indication for my section: Transverse lie.

The very first eye-contact and intensive physical contact with my second child: Approx. 20 minutes after the operation.

The Caesarean interfered with the mother-child bonding: No.

I would have preferred a natural (vaginal) birth: Yes.

I was afraid of pain during birth/of perineal trauma: No.

I was afraid of a possible Caesarean section: No.

The possibility of a Caesarean was prognosticated: Yes.

I experienced the Caesarean section as traumatic: No.

The Caesarean section was the ideal way of giving birth as far as I am concerned: No.

The birth of my third child (vaginal delivery): A beautiful birth – everything was the way I had always wanted it to be.

I find that Caesarean section is trivialised and minimised by the media (newspaper, magazines, television, …): Yes.

Due to the following the rate of Caesareans is rising: Fear of pain when giving birth, financial reasons for some gynaecologists.

My fundamental attitude on the topic "Caesarean": If the Caesarean section is absolutely necessary for medical reasons there is no doubt – then it is definitely the right and best way!

Additional notes: My aversion to having a Caesarean section was very strong. It was a longed for pregnancy and I wanted to deliver my child the "natural way". I also had misgivings that my "sleeping" during the birth could, maybe, negatively affect bonding with my child. We had agreed upon my, then 16-year old, daughter being allowed to attend the birth – because of the Caesarean this was not possible. With hindsight the whole family realised that neither bonding with the baby nor joy in the days following the birth had been negatively affected. Quite the opposite: I felt particularly wonderful, I could breastfeed immediately and the joy we felt with our baby was untroubled. My "Caesarean son" has become a very even-tempered and amazing grown-up. As a little child, though, he was a rather restless, fidgety boy who slept very fitfully for the first nine months of his life and just did not adopt a pattern. At the age of seven he was diagnosed with hyperactivity but this disappeared completely with the onset of puberty.

My Caesarean scar (length approx. 14 cm):

I massaged my scar with Saint-John's-wort oil. The scar healed fast and well, it was almost invisible by the age of about 55. I am now 57 years old and a little bulge has formed above the scar – which does not bother me though.

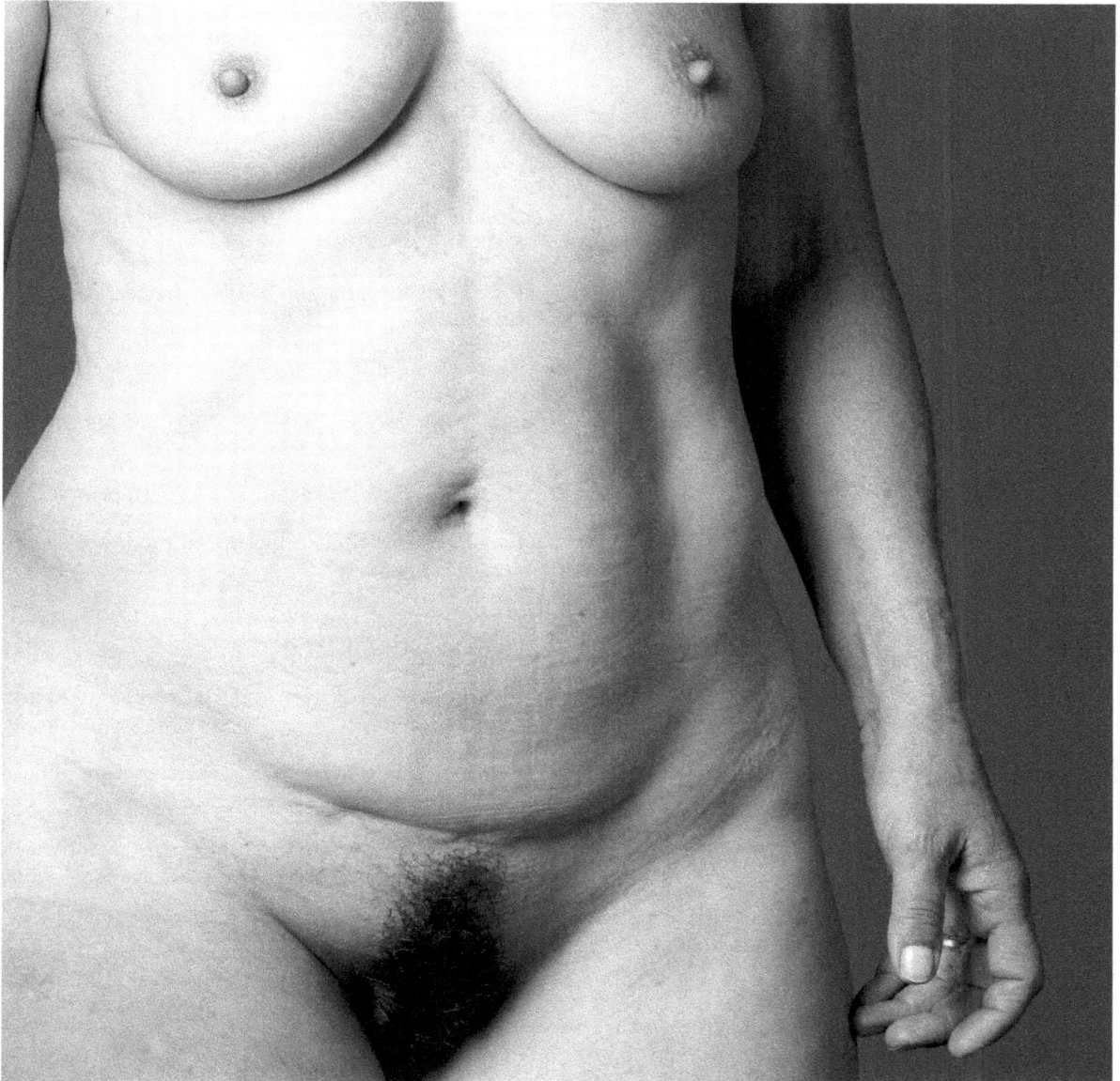

Due to the following the rate of Caesareans is rising:

At best because mothers are more self-confident and
do not let physicians talk them into things.

Occupation: At present retired, before secretary and branch manager.

When I hear the word "Caesarean section" the following words come to mind spontaneously: Breech presentation, rather large child, therefore did not want him to have to go through this complicated "exit", arranged with physician who wanted to convince me of a "normal" birth shortly beforehand, I insisted on the section, midwife discovered that the decision was right, umbilical cord was too short, cared for the child on my own from the first day without problems.

The birth of my first child (vaginal delivery): After 11 hours the question arose: Where are the extreme pains? Birth was long but easy.

The birth of my second child (vaginal delivery): 7 hours, very painful due to drip infusion.

I dealt with Caesareans intensively prior to my first Caesarean birth: No.

The birth of my third child (section): Contractions: No. Head circumference 31 cm, height 52 cm, weight 3650 g, duration of pregnancy: 40 weeks. The birth was easy for both of us.

The indication for my section: Breech presentation.

I did not receive drugs prior to the Caesarean: Waters broke shortly before, therefore just the right time.

The very first eye-contact and intensive physical contact with my child: Approx. 1 hour after the operation.

I was able to breastfeed without difficulty after the Caesarean: Yes, I breastfed for more than six months.

The Caesarean did not interfere with the mother-child bonding: The father took the baby immediately.

I would have preferred a natural (vaginal) birth: No.

I was afraid of pain during birth/of perineal trauma: No.

I was afraid of a possible Caesarean section: No.

The possibility of a Caesarean was prognosticated: No.

I miss having a natural birth experience: No.

I feel inferior due to having missed out on the experience of birth: No.

I experienced the Caesarean section as traumatic: No.

The Caesarean section was the ideal way of giving birth as far as I am concerned: No.

I think that in future Caesarean section should generally replace vaginal birth: No.

The birth of my fourth child (vaginal delivery): Just took one hour, child broke her collarbone during delivery.

My fundamental attitude on the topic "Caesarean": What has to be, has to be – period. You must approach it positively.

My Caesarean scar (length approx. ? cm):

Not visible.

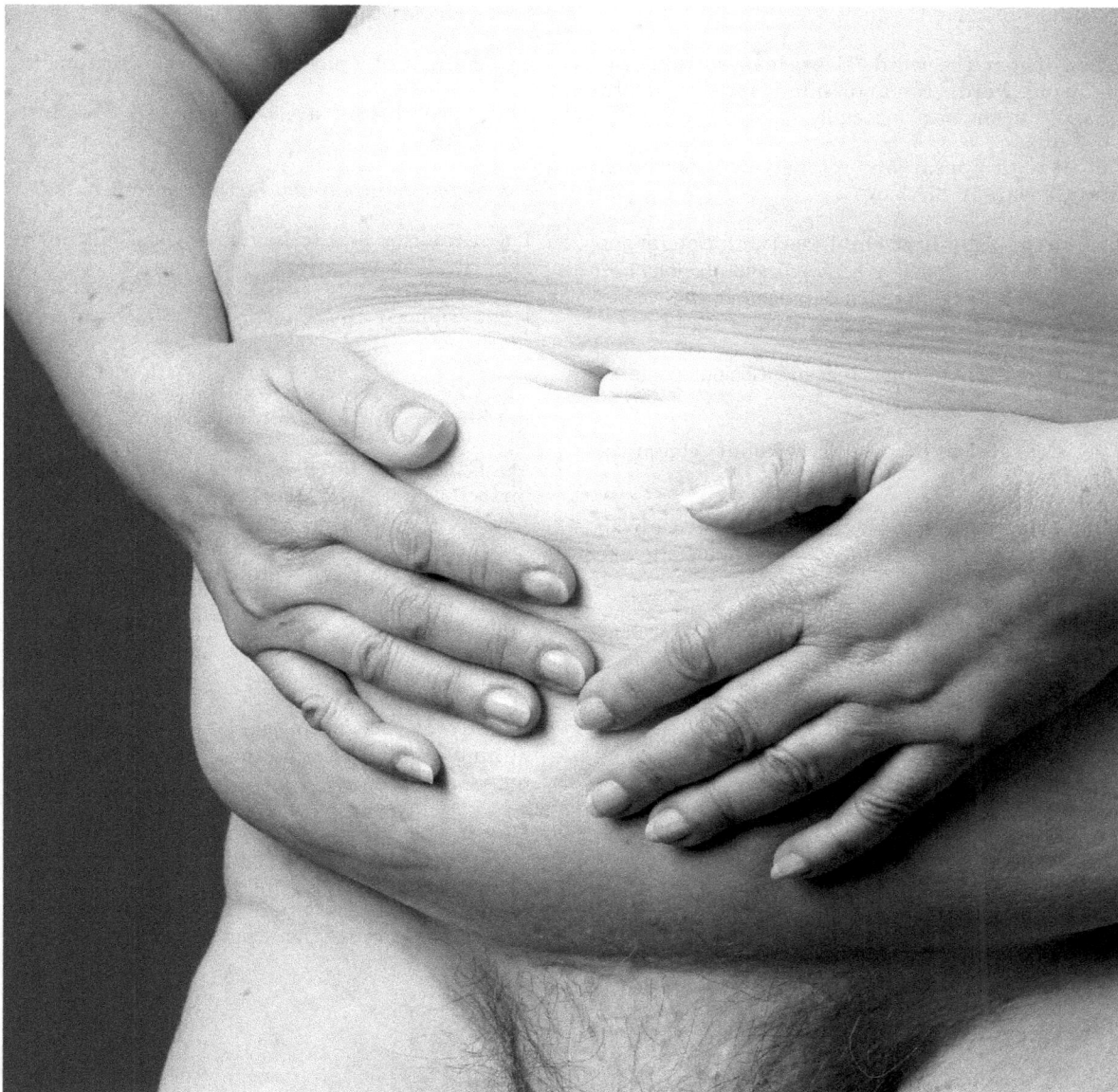

I had health problems after the Caesarean section:

I was very weak for a long time.

Occupation: Retired.

When I hear the word "Caesarean section" the following words come to mind spontaneously: Disappointment, pain, insecurity.

I dealt with Caesareans intensively prior to my first Caesarean birth: No.

The birth of my first child (section): Natural and induced labour: Altogether approx. 48 hours. Height 55 cm, weight 3500 g, duration of pregnancy: 40 weeks. Endless waiting – pain – desperation.

The indication for my section: Occiput posterior presentation.

The Caesarean proceeded without complications: Yes.

The very first eye-contact and intensive physical contact with my child: Approx. 8 hours after the operation.

I did not breastfeed after the Caesarean: Was not allowed – fever!

The Caesarean interfered with the mother-child bonding: Back then the babies were only brought for breastfeeding – I did not breastfeed and therefore hardly ever held my baby!

I would have preferred a natural (vaginal) birth: Yes.

I was afraid of pain during birth: Yes.

I was afraid of perineal trauma: No.

I was afraid of a possible Caesarean section: No.

The possibility of a Caesarean was prognosticated: Yes.

I miss having a natural birth experience: Yes.

I feel inferior due to having missed out on the experience of birth: No.

I experienced the Caesarean section as traumatic: Yes.

The Caesarean section was the ideal way of giving birth as far as I am concerned: No.

My Caesarean birth is seen as a fully-fledged birth by my family, friends and acquaintances: Yes.

Society gives me the feeling of having failed: No.

The birth of my second child (vaginal delivery): Very afraid in the beginning due to the experience of the first birth, then great relief!

I find that Caesarean section is trivialised and minimised by the media (newspaper, magazines, television, …): Yes.

Due to the following the rate of Caesareans is rising: Fear of pain during birth.

My fundamental attitude on the topic "Caesarean": Emergency solution – but not an alternative.

My Caesarean scar (length approx. 20 cm):

A straight line with visible punctures on both sides. My Caesarean scar healed without a problem. I cannot feel my Caesarean scar. It is easy for me to accept my Caesarean scar but I find it ugly.

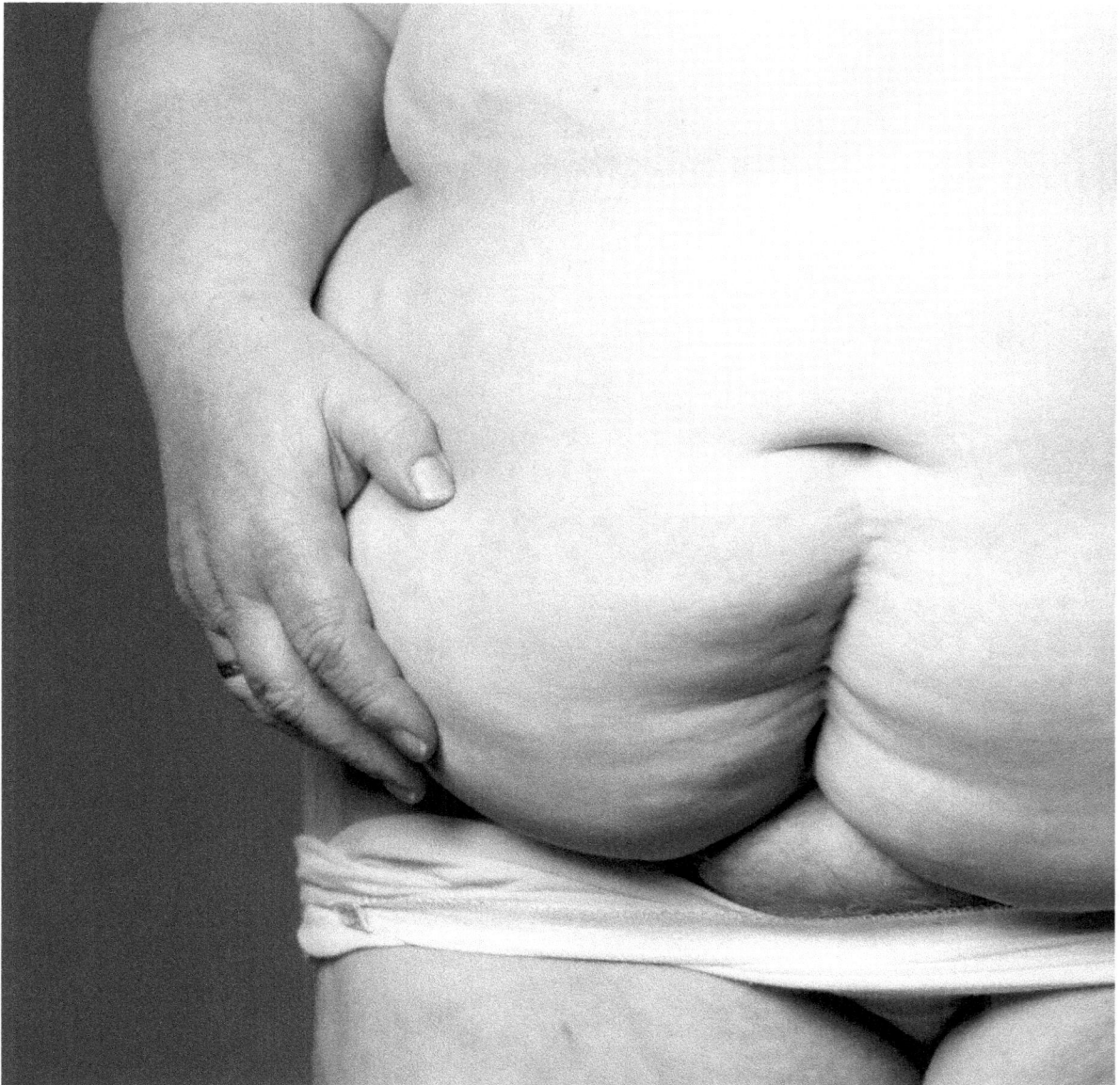

Caesarean mothers with two sections

[T010] The following complications occurred during the second Caesarean section:

Uterine atony (uterus had to be massaged as it would not contract). Through this I also lost a lot of blood. Received 3 units of blood after the birth.

Occupation: Employee. At present: Maternity leave.

When I hear the word "Caesarean section" the following words come to mind spontaneously: Pain, fear, emergency solution, complications.

The birth of my first child (first section): Natural contractions: Approx. 10 hours. Head circumference 34 cm, height 53 cm, weight 2820 g, duration of pregnancy: 36 weeks +6 days. Unfortunately, I did not read up on the topic of "sections", it was a great surprise for us.

The indication for my first section: Malposition of the child (brow presentation), fever, foetal tachycardia.

The very first eye-contact with my first child: Approx. 2 hours after the operation.

The first intensive physical contact with my first child: Approx. 10 hours after the operation.

I did not want to breastfeed after the first birth: I never breastfed.

The birth of my second child (second section): Natural contractions: Approx. 10 hours. Head circumference 36 cm, height 54 cm, weight 3800 g, duration of pregnancy: 38 weeks +6 days. It was a little more relaxed as I had an epidural during the entire birth. Despite this, it was again very unexpected.

The indication for my second section: Malposition of the child, uterine atony.

The very first eye-contact with my second child: During the operation.

The first intensive physical contact with my second child: Approx. 2 hours after the operation.

I was able to breastfeed without difficulty after the second Caesarean: I breastfed for a couple of months.

I had health problems after my second Caesarean section: Thrombosis.

I would have preferred natural (vaginal) births: Yes.

I was afraid of pain during birth/of perineal trauma: No.

I was afraid of a possible Caesarean section: No.

The possibility of a Caesarean was prognosticated both times: No.

I experienced both Caesarean sections as traumatic: No.

The Caesarean sections were the ideal way of giving birth as far as I am concerned: No.

Both my Caesarean births are seen as fully-fledged births by my family, friends and acquaintances: As I was allowed to experience everything up to the pushing contractions.

Due to the following the rate of Caesareans is rising: Fear of pain during birth and of the duration.

My fundamental attitude on the topic "Caesarean": If nothing else is possible I find it OK. (Health of mother and child has first priority.) But I would try to deliver normally every time. The Caesareans were neither fantastic deliveries nor traumatic for me. I am just happy to have "healthy" children and that it all went well for me too. If it wasn't for the Caesarean a lot would have gone wrong in my case.

My Caesarean scar (length approx. 13 cm):

Since the thrombosis I have a varicose vein next to my scar. Both my scars are just slightly apart. The second scar is a lot longer than the first. From time to time I feel a sharp pain where my Caesarean scars are when getting up or with weather changes.

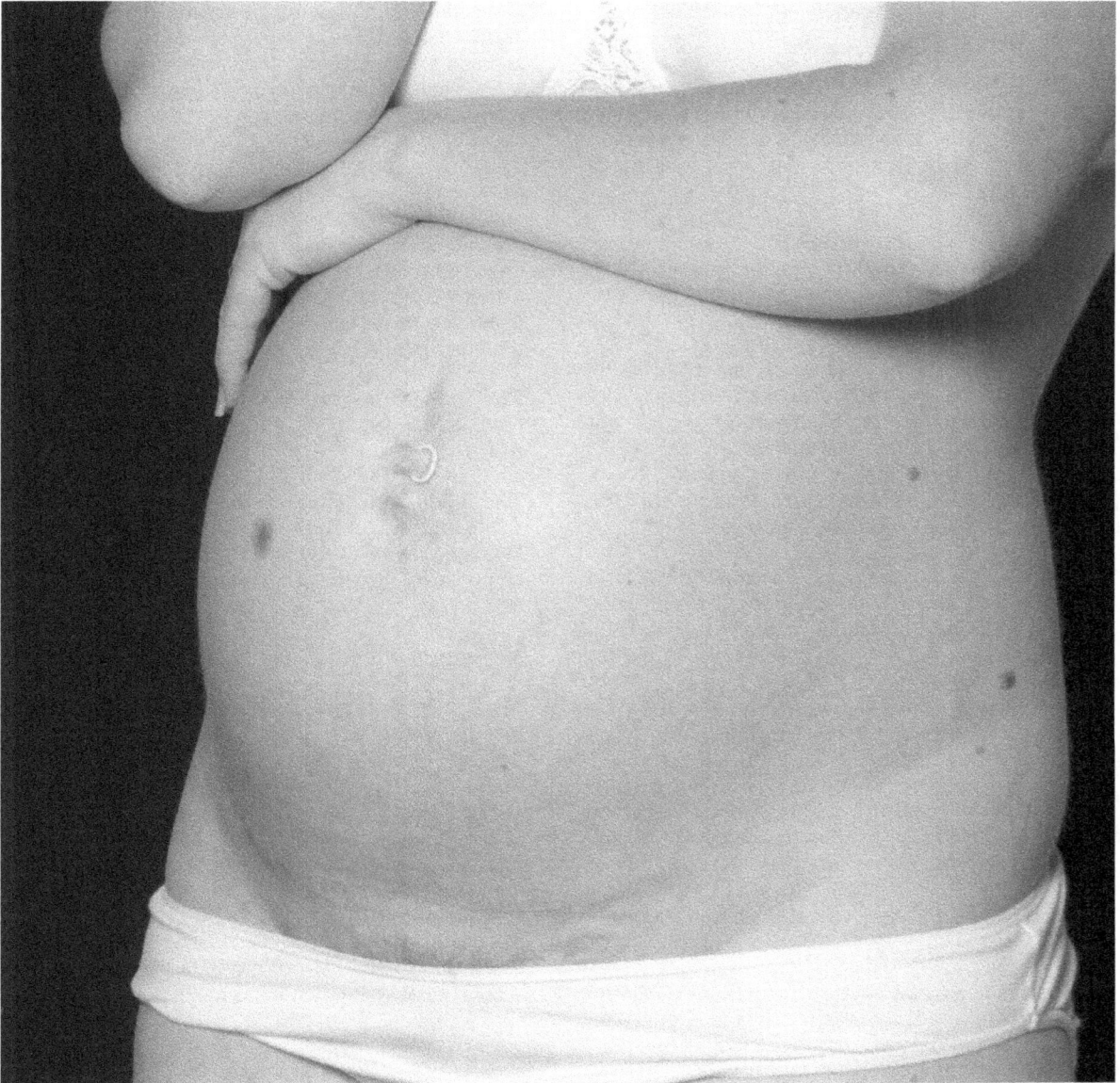

Caesarean mothers with two sections

And have the feeling of finally arriving. It is great and important that people embrace this topic in such a way that does not only show the section as being "trendy", risk-free, great, easy to schedule, manageable; but better yet, in such a way that there is not only the pain of the wound but also the very deep pain of the soul which has to heal.

Occupation: Kindergarten teacher in the field of social education.

When I hear the word "Caesarean section" the following words come to mind spontaneously: Emergency exit, sadness, being at someone's mercy, failure, I miss "holding children in my arms" and forgetting about the pain…

Caesareans were not an issue for me before my first Caesarean birth: But I always asked about it in the antenatal class. Answer: You won't have that, everybody delivers "normally".

The birth of my first child (first section): Natural contractions: Approx. 11 hours. Induced labour: Approx. 30 minutes. Head circumference 34.5 cm, height 53 cm, weight 3798 g, duration of pregnancy: 41 weeks. Horror: "Quickly the child…….sign this" – panic, hecticness, "so, now you can sleep and your baby will be delivered" – WAIT – I am not ready yet…

The indication for my first section: Discoloured amniotic fluid, failure to progress at pelvic brim, placental insufficiency (gestational diabetes type I), pathological CTG.

Prior to the first Caesarean I received drugs: Medication to speed up labour, to bring birth to an end.

The following complications occurred during the first Caesarean: My son had adaptive difficulties, had drunk discoloured amniotic fluid and had it in his lungs, child in a very bad general condition, Apgar 6-8-8. 12 hours of intensive care followed WITHOUT mum!

The first Caesarean section interfered with the mother-child bonding: Everyone (grandparents etc.) got to know Jan before I did, they brought the "fully dressed child" to me (12 hours later).

I ascribe the following peculiarities of my first child to the Caesarean birth: Difficult theory: My son had to immediately "trust" many different people – he is still extremely outgoing today and approaches people, is not shy of others.

The birth of my second child (second section): Natural contractions: Approx. 4 hours. Head circumference 35 cm, height 52 cm, weight 3450 g, duration of pregnancy: 39 ½ weeks. Inner feeling, heavy-handed unpleasant midwife – cervix had dilated 3.5 cm after 4 hours (very strong contractions every minute), "No painkillers for a vaginal delivery – you chose a section the first time"…

The indication for my second section: Scar pain (personal uneasy inner feeling), gestational diabetes type I.

The following complications occurred during the second Caesarean: Stress in the operating theatre! My daughter was unexpectedly blue, did not breathe immediately, had to be reanimated, although it was NOT an emergency Caesarean section (Apgar 2-7-9).

My second child has health problems now: No.

My family, friends and acquaintances partly give me the feeling of having failed: "It was easy for you anyway!"

Due to the following the rate of Caesareans is rising: Easy to schedule, manageable, safe, "pain free" (which painkillers do celebrities get afterwards? …)

My fundamental attitude on the topic "Caesarean": Undesirable way of giving birth, not necessary – but if it has to be then it has to be…

My Caesarean scar (length approx. 14 cm):

My torso turned into a "face": The eyes are the nipples, the navel is the nose, the scar is the mouth... My children can always have a look at "where they came from"! The scar makes me sad but gave me my two angels (without a Caesarean I would not have either of my children).

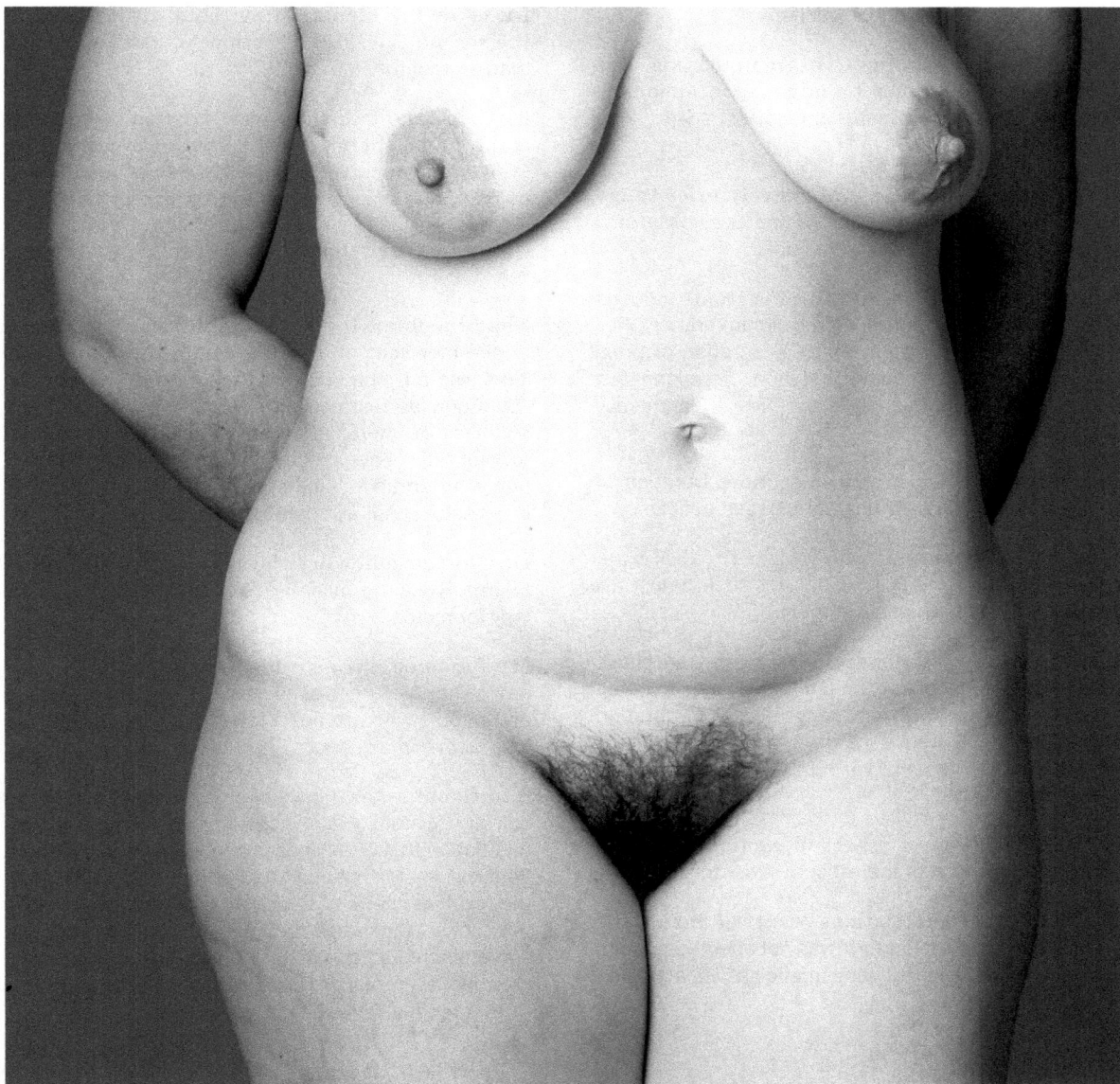

Caesarean mothers with two sections

[T147]   After my two Caesarean deliveries I have the feeling:

Of only having one "Joker" left in my hand.

Occupation: Middle school teacher.

When I hear the word "Caesarean section" the following words come to mind spontaneously: Emergency solution, unnatural, helpless, scars, dead abdomen.

I dealt with Caesareans intensively prior to my first Caesarean birth: Due to the possibility of a breech presentation with my first child.

The birth of my first child (first section): Induced labour: Approx. 15 hours. Head circumference 37.5 cm, height 52 cm, weight 3910 g, duration of pregnancy: 42 weeks. Breech presentation – rotation – two weeks overdue – induction of the birth – emergency Caesarean section.

The indication for my first section: Duration of birth too long, child suffering from oxygen deficiency.

I had problems breastfeeding after the first Caesarean section: My child could not suck properly. I breastfed for more than six months.

The birth of my second child (second section): Natural contractions: Approx. 6 hours. Head circumference 33 cm, height 50 cm, weight 3300 g, duration of pregnancy: 38 weeks +3 days. I rejected the suggestion of a delivery via vacuum extractor – elective Caesarean section???

The indication for my second section: Failure to progress – rejection of the vacuum extractor.

The following complications occurred during the second Caesarean: Epidural was not effective enough (I felt the cut) – received anaesthetic gas via a mask?

I was able to breastfeed without difficulty after the second Caesarean section: I breastfed for more than six months.

I ascribe the following peculiarities of both my children to their respective Caesarean births: Even-tempered, quiet infants, low perception of pain, no panicking when going to doctors (vaccination).

I would have preferred a natural (vaginal) birth: Yes.

I had the following health problems: After surgery on the meniscus of my left knee I had extreme problems with a lymph obstruction in my leg. Full function could only be restored after 15 lymphatic drainages. My massage therapist told me, from experience, that women often have problems with their lymphatic system after an abdominal operation with an abdominal cross-section (for example Elephantiasis).

Due to the following the rate of Caesareans is rising: Risks are minimised for children and particularly for mothers.

My fundamental attitude on the topic "Caesarean": The Caesarean section is an emergency solution and people who are not affected have no idea of the long-term consequences.

Additional notes: I have been thinking about a third delivery for four years. According to medical recommendation this is only possible one more time without health risks. My husband and I often discuss whether the right moment has arrived or if we should save this "Joker" for later. Added to which I am scared that something could go wrong after my two miscarriages (possibly even stillbirth by Caesarean section) and a further pregnancy would be impossible.

My Caesarean scars (length approx. 12 cm):

My Caesarean scars healed without a problem. I can feel my Caesarean scars.
They often itch. It is not easy for me to touch my Caesarean scars.

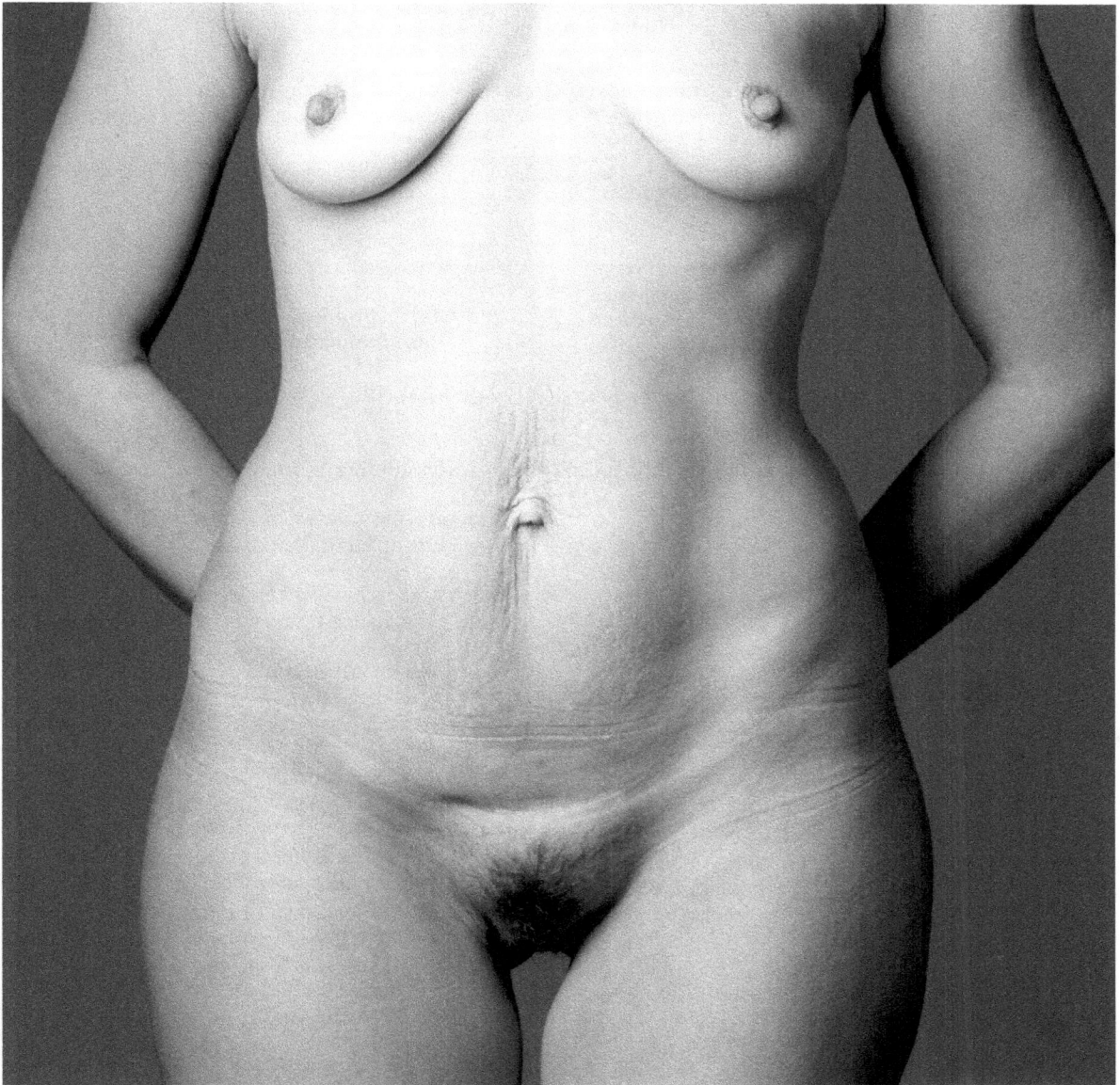

[T 150]   My husband and I, we actually wanted three children:

I don't know if and when I will be ready for a third child. The fear
of a third Caesarean section is too great at the moment. I am
taking what comes in life. Who knows what it will bring.

Occupation: Bank employee.

When I hear the word "Caesarean section" the following words come to mind spontaneously: Anxiety, pain, sadness, helpless/being at someone's mercy, anger.

I dealt with Caesareans intensively prior to my first Caesarean birth: No.

The birth of my first child (first section): Natural contractions: Approx. 9 hours. Head circumference 35.5 cm, height 52 cm, weight 3300 g, duration of pregnancy: 40 weeks +4 days.

The indication for my first section: The baby's heart tones, unfavourable cervix.

The very first eye-contact with my first child: Approx. 4 hours after the operation.

The first intensive physical contact with my first child: Approx. 7 hours after the operation.

The first Caesarean interfered with the mother-child bonding: This baby was not "my" baby, it only turned into "my baby" at home (after one week).

I had problems breastfeeding after the first Caesarean section: Not enough breast milk, after three weeks of infected nipples: weaned.

The birth of my second child (second section): Natural contractions: Approx. 12 hours. Induced labour: Approx. 3 hours. Head circumference 35 cm, height 53 cm, weight 3178 g, duration of pregnancy: 40 weeks +5 days.

The indication for my second section: The baby's heart tones, unfavourable cervix.

The very first eye-contact with my second child: During the operation.

The first intensive physical contact with my second child: Approx. 10 hours after the operation.

The second Caesarean interfered with the mother-child bonding: n.s.

I did not want to breastfeed after the second Caesarean: I did not breastfeed.

I had health problems after my second Caesarean section: Thrombosis.

I would have preferred natural (vaginal) births: Yes.

I was afraid of pain during birth: Yes.

I feel inferior due to having missed out on the experience of birth: Partially yes.

Due to the following the rate of Caesareans is rising: Trivialisation by the media.

My fundamental attitude on the topic "Caesarean": For health reasons I think it is great that the possibility exists but psychological support for the mother is forgotten!

Additional notes: Why I took so long to fill in the questionnaire: Fear of my feelings, having to "live through" the two Caesareans again. The question "why me?", "why did I have to experience this and can and what am I supposed to learn from this?" In hind-sight I am thankful for these experiences with the Caesareans, I have changed a lot because of them. And via this project I have finally dealt with and finalised this topic! – THANK YOU –

My Caesarean scar (length approx. 15,5 cm):

A short dividing line between my upper and lower body. The scar does not bother me, it healed very well and nicely, I am just reminded about it every time I take a shower. Just above the scar I have a few "numb" spots which feel "different" and which I am aware of especially before my period (light pain).

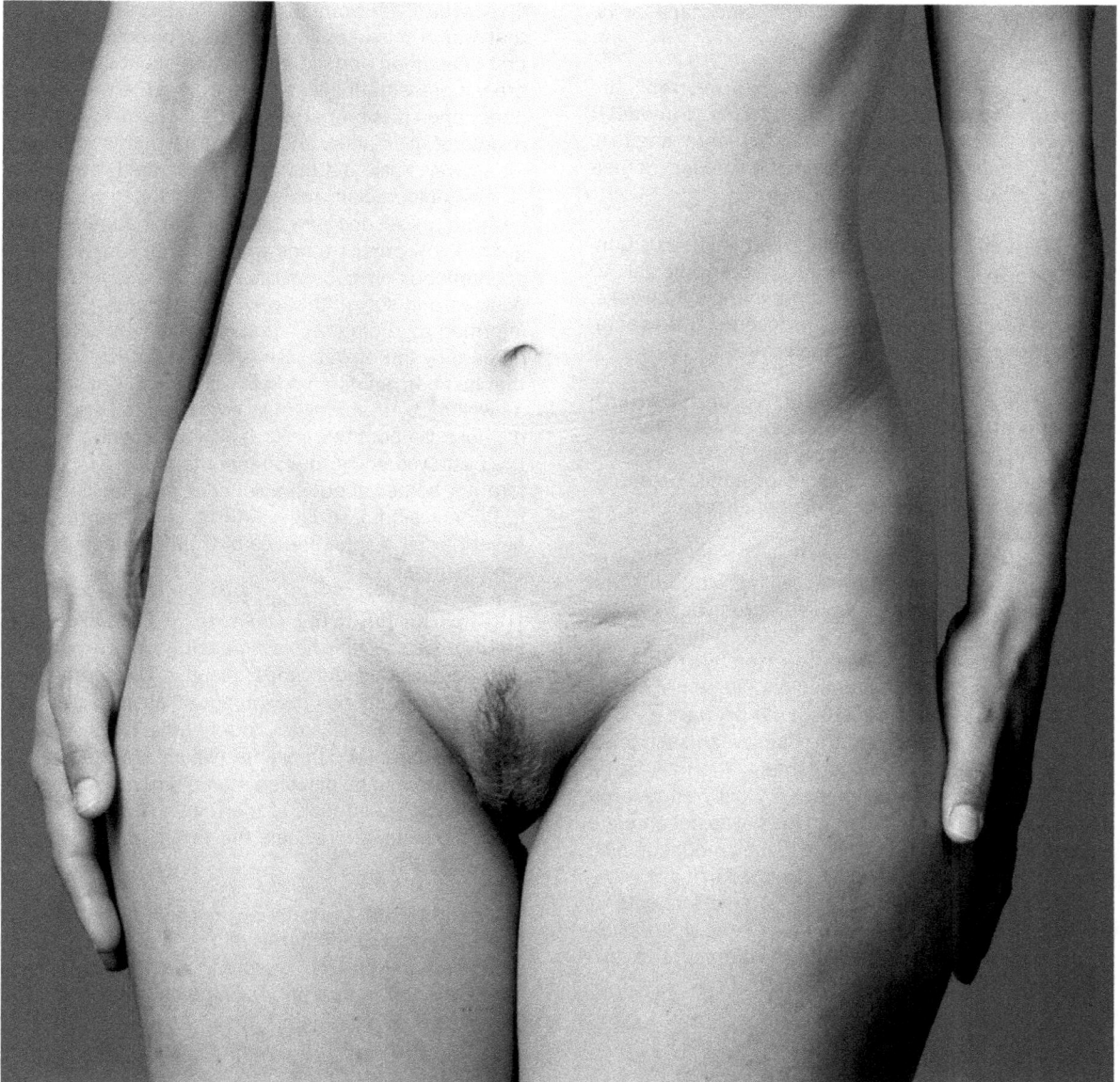

[T085] I did not waste thoughts on a repeated Caesarean during my second pregnancy:

Today I see this carelessness as a disadvantage and as a mistake as I, for example, might have chosen a different maternity clinic if I had been more aware before the second birth. Under different circumstances the birth might have proceeded in a different way? I will never know!

Occupation: Landscape gardener, landscape architect.

When I hear the word "Caesarean section" the following words come to mind spontaneously: Quick cut – long way, pain (physical), mental anguish, struggle, finality, irreversible, being at someone's mercy, envy, longing for spontaneous birth.

The birth of my first child (first section): Contractions: No. Head circumference 36 cm, height 50 cm, weight 3520 g, duration of pregnancy: 39 weeks. Planned Caesarean section due to breech presentation, positive memories, no complications.

The birth of my second child (second section): Natural contractions: Approx. 12 hours. Head circumference 35 cm, height 55 cm, weight 4070 g, duration of pregnancy: 41 weeks. Occiput posterior presentation, failure to progress (head did not engage.)

I suffered from depression after the second Caesarean: Sense of inferiority, struggling with the situation, envying other women who delivered vaginally.

I had problems breastfeeding after both Caesarean sections: Not enough milk: supplementary feeding. I do not ascribe the fact that I did not have enough milk (with both children) to the Caesarean section(s)! I never had the classic engorgement, the milk came slowly and without problems but my children just did not get enough i.e. the following meal was not enough. I left no stone unturned to increase the amount of milk: different globules, lactation oil, lemonade on a milk basis (a Swiss drink called "Rivella"), large amounts of tea etc. At one point, in both cases, it seemed to be wise to alternate the bottle and the breast to relieve me from stress. I enjoyed breastfeeding.

Caesarean sections did not matter to me: And that was a mistake! I was totally clueless before the first Caesarean and did not read up about it at all. The breech presentation was there during the whole pregnancy and I was prepared for a Caesarean. I was in the middle of my studies and did not have time to think a lot anyway. I also did not get any informative tips from others (obstetrician, midwives, friends). It was different with my second pregnancy, in the meantime I had got to know other women with children and wanted a spontaneous birth. Soon my daughter was in the right position and stayed that way. Unfortunately, I was not informed regarding my situation (condition after Caesarean) by the obstetrician (who also forgot to tell me that he does not do epidurals with repeat Caesareans) as well as by the midwife in the antenatal class, who did not talk about this topic at all. I was totally sure that the birth was going to work spontaneously, did therefore not bother about special care or a special clinic! [...] Conclusion: I struggle with my situation (possibly never having a spontaneous birth) more because I reproach myself.

Due to the following the rate of Caesareans is rising: Obstetricians have increasingly less experience with complicated deliveries, elective Caesarean sections: women choose the supposed easier way which is also so wonderfully easy to schedule, physicians are afraid of parent's complaints (which are increasing), should the child be disabled after a difficult vaginal delivery. The presentation of the Caesarean section e.g. in public (celebs) conceals the fact that it is surgery with all its risks.

My fundamental attitude on the topic "Caesarean": They cut too fast, the mother's psyche is totally disregarded. With the Caesarean section one misses out on the experience of bringing a child into the world using one's own strength.

33 years • S:SPA [27, g] • S:SPA [31, g] {14th week of pregnancy, the baby girl was delivered vaginally}

My Caesarean scar (length approx. 13.5 cm):

During menstruation or during ovulation I sometimes feel a dragging pain. It is not a problem for me to accept my scar (as opposed to my two Caesareans), for both my children this was their way into life!

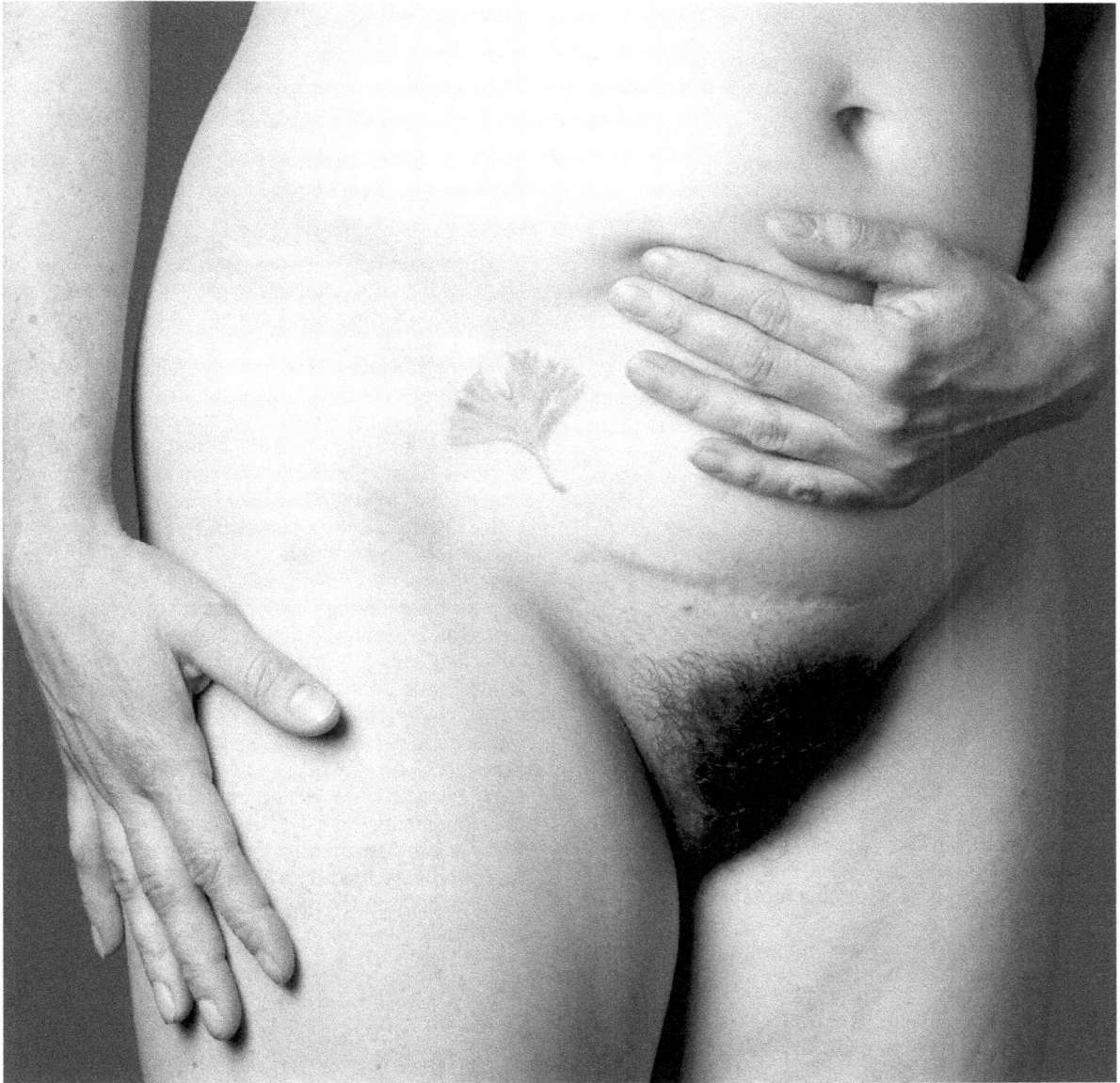

[T057] The second Caesarean section proceeded without complications:

Complications were avoided by the Caesarean. During surgery an undiagnosed uterine rupture was discovered.

Occupation: Executive / Personality counsellor.

When I hear the word "Caesarean section" the following words come to mind spontaneously: Baby, surgery, abdomen, cut, hospital.

I dealt with Caesareans intensively prior to my first Caesarean birth: Breech presentation, my physician let me decide all by myself. A vaginal birth was too risky for me. I was not influenced although my physician is part of a special team for vaginal breech births.

The birth of my first child (first section): Natural Contractions: No, although the CTG showed effective contractions the morning of the surgery. Head circumference 37.5 cm, height 48 cm, weight 3410 g, duration of pregnancy: 38 weeks +4 days. Planned Caesarean section 10 days before term because of breech presentation.

I was able to breastfeed without difficulty after the first Caesarean: I breastfed for more than half a year.

I might ascribe the following peculiarities of my first child to the Caesarean birth: A colicky baby.

The birth of my second child (second section): Natural contractions: No, but CTG regularly every 7 minutes (premonitory pains). Head circumference 38 cm, height 49 cm, weight 3300 g, duration of pregnancy: 36 weeks +4 days. Planned Caesarean section, readjusted near-term 3 weeks earlier because of a very large head. Undiagnosed uterine rupture.

The indication for my second section: Very large head and previous Caesarean.

I was able to breastfeed without difficulty after the second Caesarean: I am still breastfeeding.

The very first eye-contact with both my children: During the operation.

The first intensive physical contact with both my children: Approx. 30 minutes after the operation.

The Caesarean section was the ideal way of giving birth as far as I am concerned: Yes

My fundamental attitude on the topic "Caesarean": I would not have chosen it but it was ideal for me. I think that a difficult vaginal delivery would have adversely affected the relationship with my child.

Additional notes: The topic "Caesarean section" causes a very controversial discussion with (expectant) mothers. On the one hand they say: You are taking the easy way out. On the other hand the Caesarean section is said to be as painful as hell. Everybody is for equality but, despite this has her own opinion. Often women who experienced the Caesarean section as traumatic are preoccupied with this topic. There is little room for positive experiences. Anyway, I know a lot more women who have had positive or neutral experiences with Caesareans and traumatic vaginal deliveries, than the other way round. In my specific case the medical advice to have Caesarean sections saved me from difficult, maybe traumatic births (breech presentation with a head circumference of 37.5 or 38 cm and undiagnosed rupture). The second birth could have ended really badly if I had waited for real contractions and full term. I think the big difference in the experience is whether the Caesarean was planned and, thereby, at least partly decided on by the woman, or if an emergency occurs during birth – fear and panic arise and there is no choice in the end.

My Caesarean scar (length approx. 14 cm):

My Caesarean scar healed without a problem, I do not feel it. After the first Caesarean the scar was hardly visible. It is still too early to tell but at the moment only slightly red. The changed feeling of my abdomen is due more to flabby abdominal muscles.

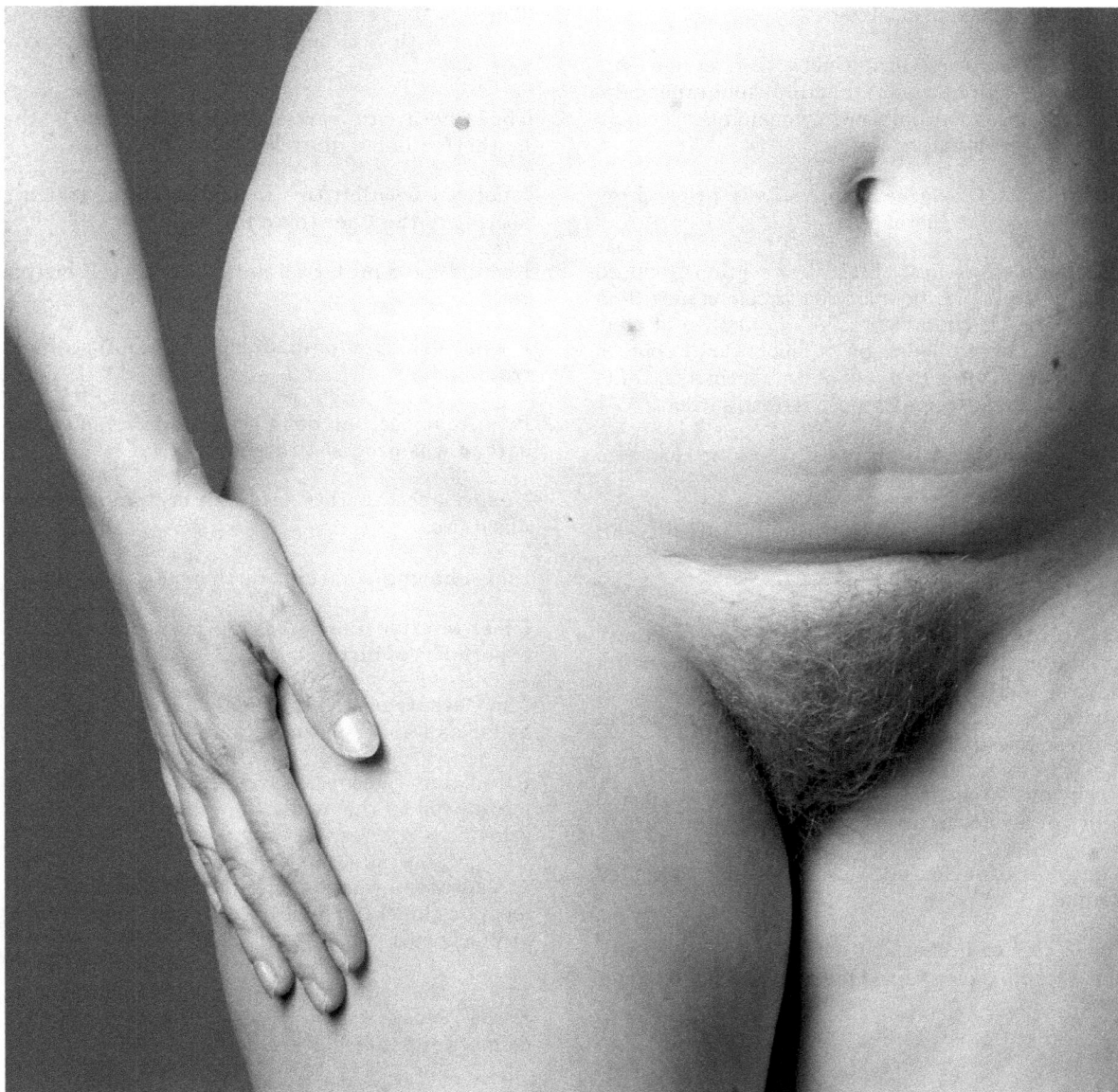

[T103] My fundamental attitude on the topic "Caesarean":

Caesarean section only if it is unavoidable for medical reasons.
A natural birth is definitely best for mother and child.

Occupation: Commercial clerk.

When I hear the word "Caesarean section" the following words come to mind spontaneously: Wound pain, abdominal section, unnatural, relief (from labour pains), lifesaving.

I dealt with Caesareans intensively prior to my first Caesarean birth: No.

The birth of my first child (first section): Induced labour: Approx. 16 hours. Head circumference 34.5 cm, height 56 cm, weight 3950 g, duration of pregnancy: 40 weeks. Induction of labour due to breech presentation. After 16 hours of contractions failure to progress (pelvis too narrow): Caesarean section.

The indication for my first section: Failure to progress with breech presentation.

I was able to breastfeed without difficulty after the first Caesarean: I breastfed for more than 1 year.

The birth of my second child (second section): Contractions: No. Head circumference 36 cm, height 55 cm, weight 4500 g, duration of pregnancy: 39 weeks. Planned Caesarean section due to a pelvis that is too narrow (and again breech presentation).

Prior to my second Caesarean section the possibility of a Caesarean was prognosticated: Yes.

The indication for my second section: Pelvis too narrow.

I was able to breastfeed without difficulty after the second Caesarean: I breastfed for more than 1 year.

The very first eye-contact and intensive physical contact with both my children: During the operation.

The Caesarean sections interfered with the mother-child bonding: No.

I noticed peculiarities in my children, which I ascribe to the Caesarean birth: No.

I would have preferred natural (vaginal) births: Yes.

I was afraid of pain during birth/of perineal trauma: No.

Prior to my second birth the possibility of a Caesarean was prognosticated: Yes.

I experienced both Caesarean sections as traumatic: No.

I miss having a natural birth experience: Yes.

I feel inferior due to having missed out on the experience of birth: No.

The Caesarean was the ideal way of giving birth as far as I am concerned: No.

I find that Caesarean section is trivialised and minimised by the media (newspaper, magazines, television, ...): Yes.

A Caesarean section possibly has negative effects on the child: If the child is "pulled out" without contractions or without prior notice.

Due to the following the rate of Caesareans is rising: Because many people think they can save themselves from the pain and the hard work.

My Caesarean scars (length approx. 8 cm):

I had my scars treated with acupuncture so that the energy can flow again.

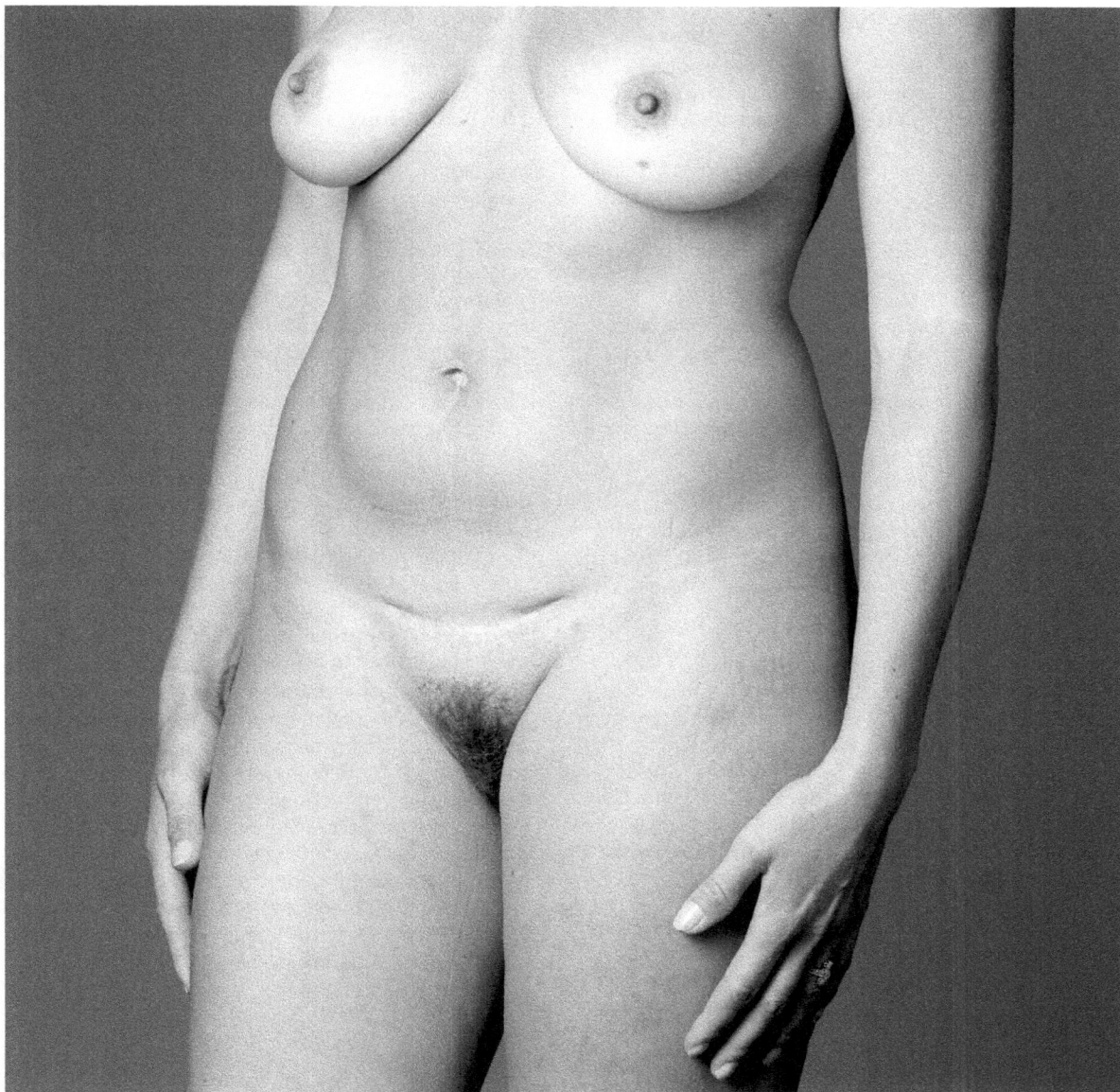

[T064] A Caesarean birth possibly has negative effects on the child:

I think that a "transitional period" is important for the baby. During labour it realises: Something is happening now, something is going to change.

Occupation: Employee (organising events).

When I hear the word "Caesarean section" the following words come to mind spontaneously: Surgery, baby, birth, anaesthesia, how unfortunate.

The birth of my first child (first section): Natural Contractions: Approx. 23 hours. Head circumference 36 cm, height 51 cm, weight 3570 g, duration of pregnancy 39 weeks +6 days. Trouble-free as such but very long first stage of labour.

The indication for my first section: Exhaustion, vacuum extraction failed, emergency section.

The very first eye-contact and intensive physical contact with my first child: Approx. 20 hours after the operation.

The first Caesarean interfered with the mother-child bonding: When I came into the postnatal ward the day after the delivery it was incredibly sad for me to see all the other mothers hugging their babies and I had not even seen my baby yet.

My first child was injured during birth: Firstly – very deformed head, secondly – scratch on the head caused by being stuck at the pubic bone and from trying to pull him out with the vacuum extractor.

My first child had serious health problems: Not because of the Caesarean, this should have been done a lot earlier; respiratory mask, asphyxia/hypoxia/cyanosis – neonatal ward.

I ascribe the following peculiarities of my first child to the Caesarean birth: "Zipper syndrome" – a year later on a camping holiday he reacted with fright when opening the tent (sound). My child has often had difficulties with "transitions": starting kindergarten, schooling; might have a connection with the Caesarean section.

The birth of my second child (second section): Natural contractions: Approx 6 hours. Head circumference 36 cm, height 54 cm, weight 3870 g, duration of pregnancy: 40 weeks +6 days.

The indication for my second section: "Stargazer", failure to progress.

I was able to breastfeed without difficulty after the second Caesarean: I am still breastfeeding.

The very first eye-contact with my second child: During the operation.

The first intensive physical contact with my second child: Approx. 1 ½ hours after the operation.

Additional notes: When I requested a Caesarean during my first delivery due to exhaustion and failure to progress, I was offered a vacuum extraction to spare me a Caesarean. I allowed myself to be persuaded, which proved wrong in the end, I could have spared my child the neonatal ward and myself the separation from him in the beginning. In my opinion I was really well prepared for my second birth using acupuncture, osteopathy and attending antenatal classes. I could again not deliver "normally". A few weeks ago I had the intrauterine contraceptive device inserted, which was very difficult according to my gynaecologist – everything is hardened, narrow and I have a bend in the uterus too. It is, therefore, quite possible that something is anatomically "different" with me. Whatever it was, this time I did not dwell on the birth for such a long time.

My Caesarean scar (length approx. 13 cm):

After the first as well as the second Caesarean section: Pain in the beginning, later itching and numbness for quite a while. The suture is not perfect, it could be more even.

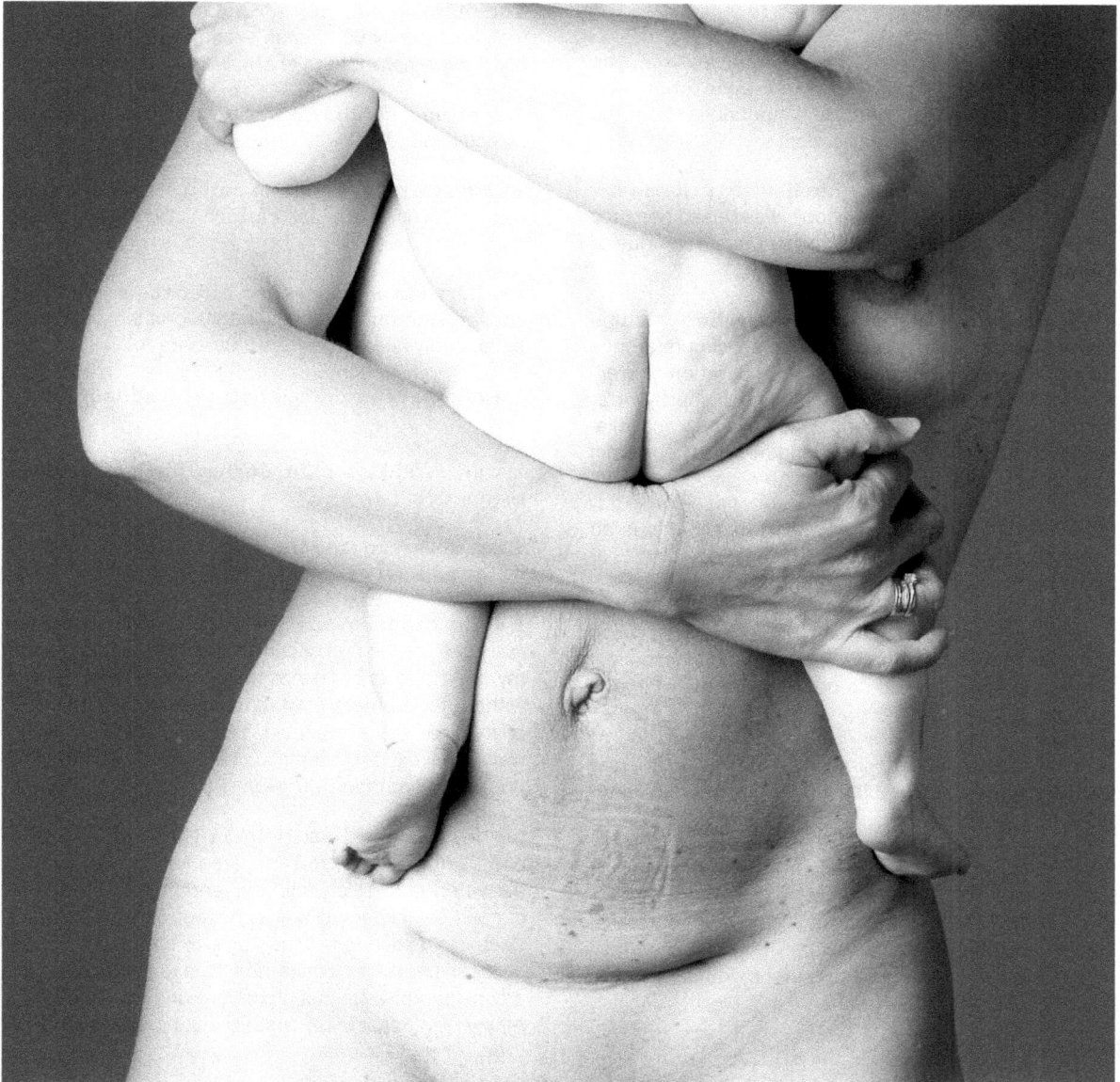

Caesarean mothers with two sections

After the first section did not feel the urge to urinate for about six months. After the second section a badly healed scar.

Occupation: Employee.

When I hear the word "Caesarean section" the following words come to mind spontaneously: Painless, security (for the child), numbness (from the waist down), surgery, complication.

I dealt with Caesareans intensively prior to my first Caesarean birth: The topic was raised because my sister delivered her first child by Caesarean due to her narrow pelvis.

The birth of my first child (first section): Natural contractions: Approx. 12 hours. Head circumference 35 cm, height 50 cm, weight 3410 g, duration of pregnancy: 41 weeks. Normal labour onset shortly after midnight. Strong contractions but delayed cervical dilatation, child squeezed against bladder, "slid" upwards: Emergency Caesarean section at 10 o'clock.

The indication for my first section: Infant's head squeezed against the bladder and she did not move or could not move anymore.

The first Caesarean section proceeded without complications: Actually yes, but they had to work very slowly and accurately so as not to injure the mother's bladder.

I suffered from depression after the first Caesarean section: Health problems (long recovery), bladder problems.

The birth of my second child (second section): Contractions: No. Head circumference 35 cm, height 51 cm, weight 3230 g, duration of pregnancy: 39 weeks. Due to the diagnosis "narrow pelvis" conscious decision to have a planned Caesarean – epidural again.

The indication for my second section: "Narrow pelvis", emergency Caesarean section with the first delivery – did not want to take any risks.

My second child had serious health problems: Difficulties breathing shortly after birth.

The very first eye-contact and intensive physical contact with both my children: During the operation.

I suffered from depression after the second Caesarean section: Caused by health problems again (fatigue, badly healed scar after Caesarean).

I would have preferred natural (vaginal) births: Yes.

I was afraid of pain during birth/of perineal trauma: No.

The Caesarean was the ideal way of giving birth as far as I am concerned: No.

Due to the following the rate of Caesareans is rising: After the first section my physician told me that my child and I would not have survived the delivery without this surgery. First reason: Nowadays, this form of medical aid is available. Secondly: Women do not want to take a risk if complications are anticipated (e.g. breech presentation). Thirdly: "Painless" birth (???)

My fundamental attitude on the topic "Caesarean": Primarily I see the Caesarean section as medical aid when mother or child are endangered. If complications are expected with a further birth, an elective Caesarean section is acceptable in terms of a healthy child, as far as I am concerned. Due to the fact that it is a considerable surgical procedure and due to the long recovery (at least in my case) I would prefer vaginal delivery if I could choose.

My Caesarean scar (length approx. 13 cm):

I never understood why celebrities insist on an elective Caesarean section for "beauty issues". Sometimes my scar bothers me, sometimes not at all. When I think of having delivered two healthy children this question is irrelevant.

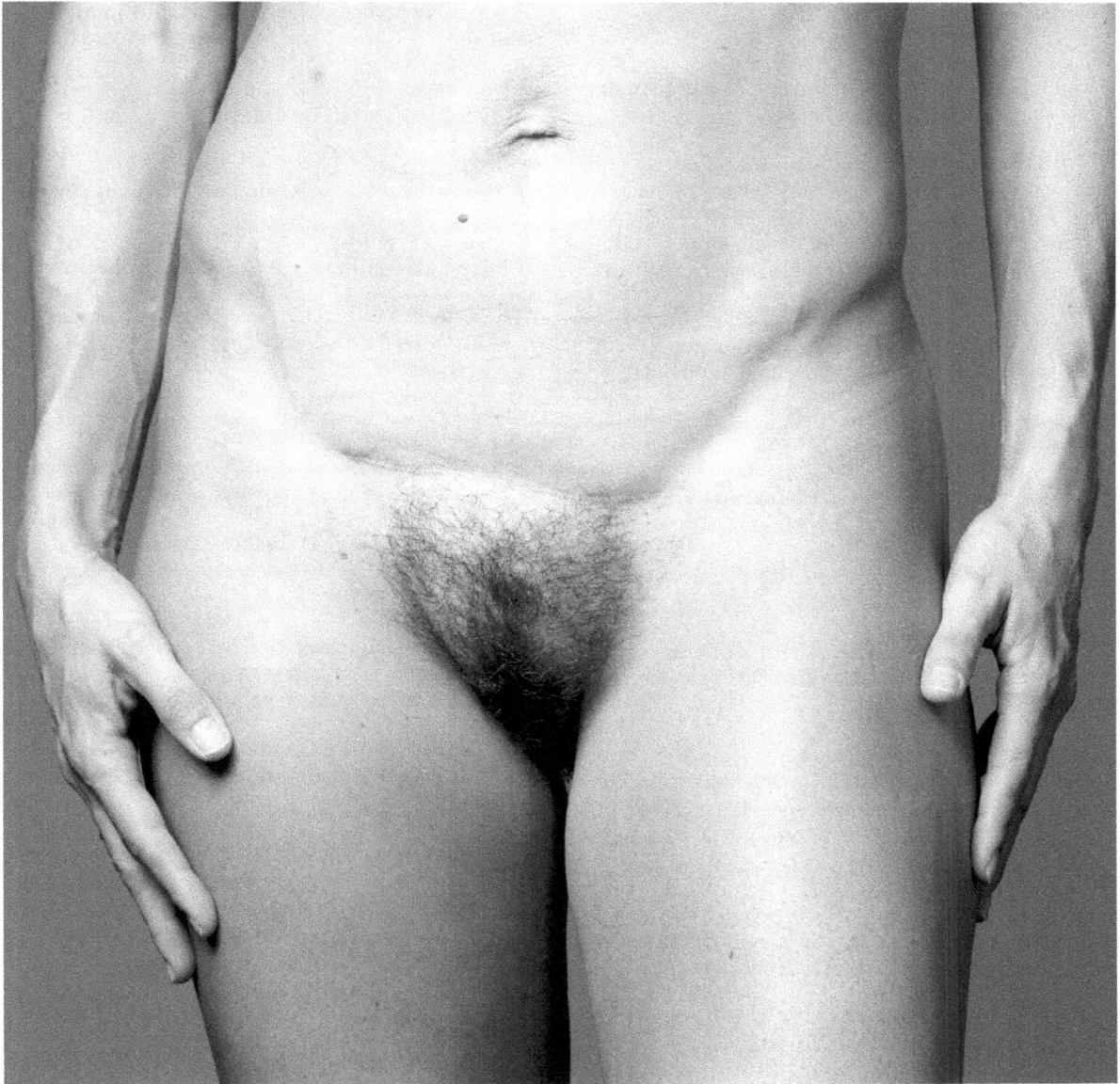

I desperately wanted to experience "normal" birth. I cannot understand how one/a woman can plan a C-Section. I tried everything to deliver without a section – but my body just did not want to play along.

Occupation: Advertising expert.

When I hear the word "Caesarean section" the following words come to mind spontaneously: Pain, scar, birth, fatigue, yearning.

The birth of my first child (first section): Natural contractions: Approx. 17 hours. Induced labour: Approx. 7 hours. Head circumference 36 cm, height 52 cm, weight 3820 g, duration of pregnancy: 42 weeks. Difficult birth, long duration, healthy child, mother feeling "off-colour".

The indication for my first section: Inadequate contractions, umbilical cord wrapped around twice.

The very first eye-contact with my first child: Approx. 1 hour after the operation.

The first intensive physical contact with my first child: Approx. 3 hours after the operation.

My first child had serious health problems after birth: Breathing.

I was able to breastfeed without difficulty after the first Caesarean: I breastfed for more than six months.

The birth of my second child (second section): Natural contractions: Approx. 2 hours. Induced labour: Approx. 6 hours. Head circumference 35 cm, height 50 cm, weight 3260 g, duration of pregnancy: 42 weeks. "Tried everything", despite this – C-section, healthy child, happy mother.

The indication for my second section: Inadequate contractions/failure to progress, delayed dilatation.

The very first eye-contact and intensive physical contact with my second child: During the operation.

I was able to breastfeed without difficulty after the second Caesarean: I breastfed for more than six months.

I would have preferred natural (vaginal) births: Yes.

I was afraid of pain during birth/of perineal trauma: No.

I miss having a natural birth experience: Yes.

The Caesarean births were the ideal way of giving birth as far as I am concerned: No.

In future Caesarean section should generally replace vaginal birth: No!

I have been having health problems since my Caesarean sections: Numbness around the scar.

I find that Caesarean section is trivialised and minimised by the media (newspaper, magazines, television, ...): Yes.

Due to the following the rate of Caesareans is rising: People want to "play it safe", with this method, obstetricians feel more important than midwives.

My fundamental attitude on the topic "Caesarean": If need be! Rather a healthy child, woman will recover...

Additional notes: It was great to deal with the births again after 6 and 3 ½ years respectively! Positive factor is: My son and I are healthy today and I was also able to give birth to my daughter thanks to the C-section!

My Caesarean scar (length approx. 14 cm):

In the meantime, it is easy for me to accept my Caesarean scar. It is fading slightly, like the pain that is and was connected with it. The marks above and below the scar, where the wound was stapled are almost more visible than the scar itself.

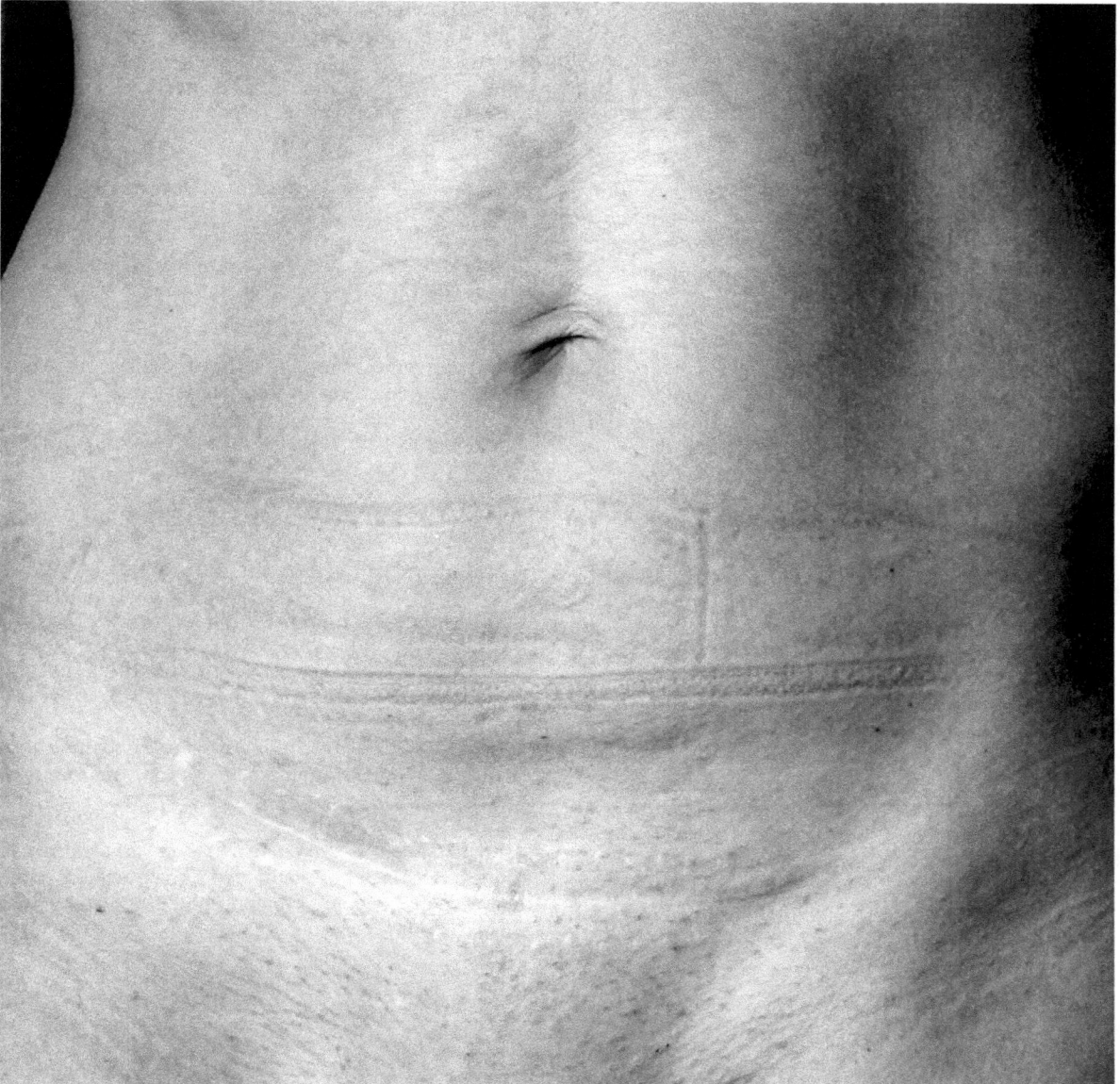

My fundamental attitude on the topic "Caesarean":

Good that the possibility exists – better still if a woman does not need it.

Occupation: Graduate social worker.

When I hear the word "Caesarean section" the following words come to my mind spontaneously: Incision, fear, "necessary", operation, being at someone's mercy.

The birth of my first child (first section): Natural contractions: Approx. 8 hours. Head circumference 36 cm, height 50 cm, weight 3550 g, duration of pregnancy: 39 weeks +6 days. Planned Caesarean section one day before term, my first hospitalisation.

The indication for my first section: Suspected cephalopelvic disproportion. Uterine fibroid.

The following complications occurred during the first Caesarean section: Heavy blood loss.

The very first eye-contact with my first child: During the operation.

The first intensive physical contact with my first child: Approx. 30 minutes after the operation.

I had problems breastfeeding after the first Caesarean: Postpartum breast engorgement took quite a while. I breastfed for more than six months.

The birth of my second child (second section): Contractions: No. Head circumference 35 cm, height 49 cm, weight 3310 g, duration of pregnancy: 38 weeks. Planned Caesarean section 10 days before term – not as bad as my first Caesarean.

The indication for my second section: Previous Caesarean section.

The following complications occurred during the first Caesarean section: Circulatory problems, heavy blood loss.

The very first eye-contact with my second child: During the operation.

The first intensive physical contact with my second child: Approx. 1 hour after the operation.

I was able to breastfeed without difficulty after the second Caesarean: Yes. I breastfed for more than six months.

I have been having health problems since my Caesarean sections: Intestinal problems.

I would have preferred natural (vaginal) births: Yes.

I was afraid of pain during birth: Yes.

I was afraid of perineal trauma: No.

I miss having a natural birth experience: Yes.

The Caesarean section was the ideal way of giving birth as far as I am concerned: No.

I find that Caesarean section is trivialised and minimised by the media (newspaper, magazines, television, ...): Yes.

Due to the following the rate of Caesareans is rising: Birth can be "planned" by obstetricians, financial reasons, women's uncertainty, in case of risk – quicker section.

My Caesarean scar (length approx. 16 cm):

Straight with two branches. Long numb zone. Sensitive skin and
tissue. I treated my scar with scar ointment and had energy blockages
unlocked. It is not easy for me to accept my Caesarean scar.

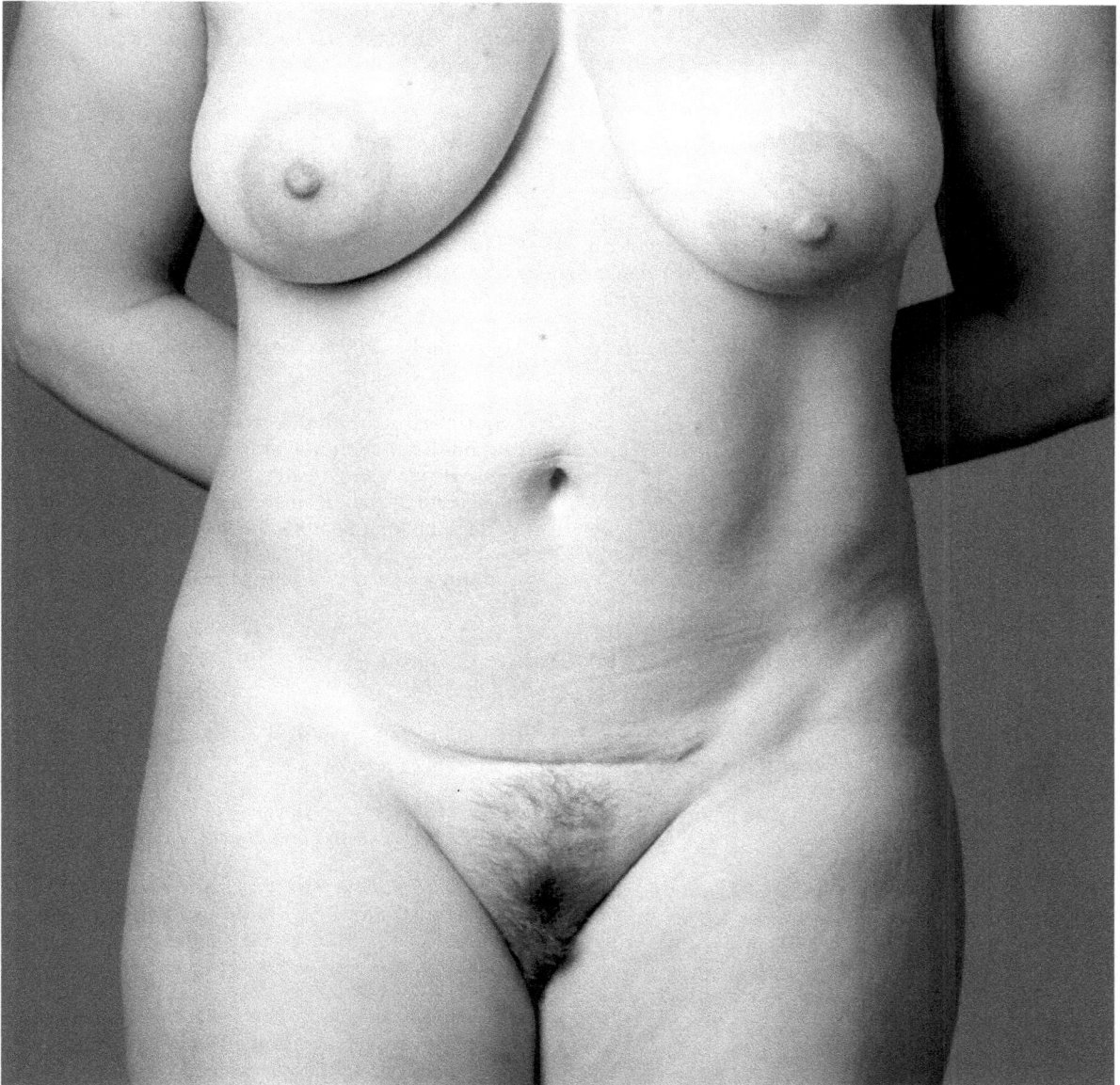

[T114]   The Caesarean section is an operation:

Every operation is dangerous and should not be trivialised. It took
me very long to have a normal perception of my body again!

Occupation: Registered health care nurse.

When I hear the word "Caesarean section" the following words come to mind spontaneously: Exhaustion, disappointment, wanting to be brave, feeling strange, failure ...

The birth of my first child (first section): Natural contractions: Approx. 10 hours. Induced labour: Approx. 9 hours. Head circumference 38 cm, height 55 cm, weight 3982 g, duration of pregnancy: 44 weeks. The lucky one. We had to get to know each other first.

The indication for my first section: Failure to progress.

The very first eye-contact with my first child: Approx. 2 hours after the operation.

The first intensive physical contact with my first child: The following morning, approx. 6 hours after the operation.

I had problems breastfeeding after the first Caesarean: I breastfed solely for 6 months, my first son was a "colicky baby" – he was hungry, didn't gain enough weight, as soon as he was given formula he was satisfied and content.

The first Caesarean interfered with the mother-child bonding: I could barely hold my son because of severe abdominal pain. He cried a lot and I was not able to calm him down.

The birth of my second child (second section): Contractions: No. Head circumference 36 cm, height 52 cm, weight 3650 g, duration of pregnancy: 36 weeks. The "worrier". You turned without anyone noticing in the last few days, so that I feel good about the second Caesarean.

The indication for my second section: Planned section due to the first birth and my physical problems afterwards.

The very first eye-contact and intensive physical contact with my second child: During the operation.

I had problems breastfeeding after the second Caesarean: My milk seems to be of "poor content". I breastfed for six months giving him the bottle afterwards.

My second child has health problems: He has sensitive skin.

I had health problems after or I have been having health problems since my Caesarean sections: Heavy bleeding after the first Caesarean, since the second Caesarean menstruation is very long, 10 to 14 days, but only spotting the last days.

I would have preferred natural (vaginal) births: Yes.

I was afraid of pain during birth/of perineal trauma: No.

I miss having a natural birth experience: No, not anymore.

The Caesarean section was the ideal way of giving birth as far as I am concerned: No.

My Caesarean births are seen as fully-fledged births by my family, friends and acquaintances: I think so, but I would not care if someone else (friends) sees my birth experiences as not being fully-fledged.

Due to the following the rate of Caesareans is rising: Because it is presented by the media and also exemplified by celebrities.

My Caesarean scar (length approx. 15 cm):

My abdominal wall around the scar feels like a huge bruise, sensitive to pressure, delicate. It feels like the scar divides my abdomen into two halves, intensified by this "bruised feeling".

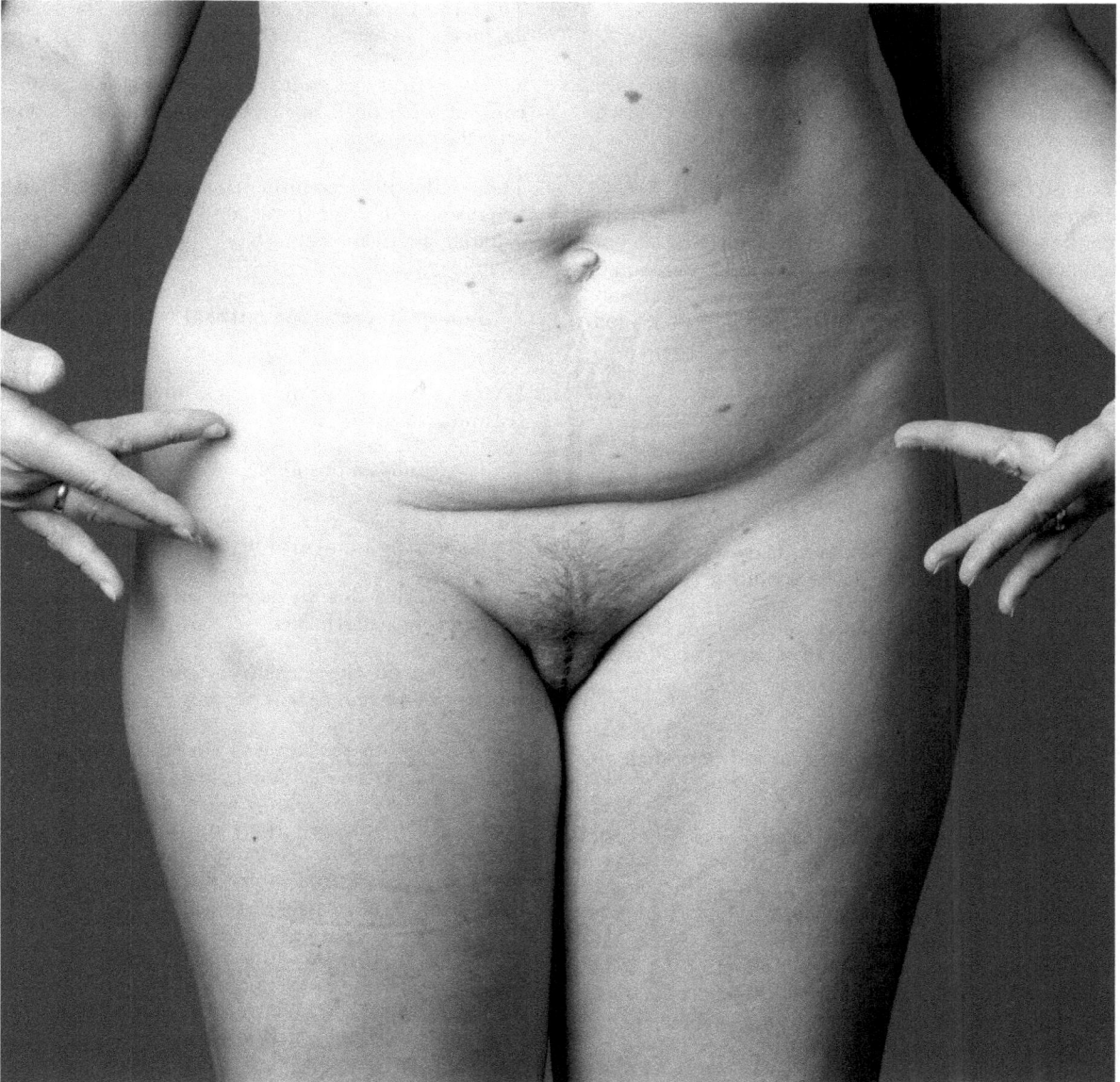

I suffered from depression after the second Caesarean section:

I will not make it, I cannot breastfeed...

Occupation: Psychologist, trainer.

When I hear the word "Caesarean section" the following words come to mind spontaneously: Scar, pain, no "real" birth, thereby healthy children, heard no first cry.

The birth of my first child (first section): Natural contractions: Approx. 23 hours. Intensified contractions due to medication: Approx. 5 hours. Head circumference n.s., height 56 cm, weight 3500 g, duration of pregnancy: 40 weeks. It was not a planned Caesarean, after 23 hours of labour an emergency Caesarean section saved the child's life.

The indication for my first section: Head too large, child did not drop into the birth canal.

The very first eye-contact with my first child: Approx. 1 hour after the operation.

The first intensive physical contact with my first child: Approx. 9 hours after the operation.

I suffered from depression after the first Caesarean: Being bound to my bed and not being able to care for my baby immediately.

I was able to breastfeed without difficulty after the first Caesarean: I breastfed for more than six months.

My first child has health problems now: Epilepsy.

The birth of my second and third child (twins, second section): Contractions: No. Head circumference n.s., height 47/48 cm, weight 2002/2998 g, duration of pregnancy: 39 weeks. The first of the twins was in a transverse position and weighed only 2 kg. The second twin was a normal baby weighing 3 kg.

The indication for my second section: Transverse lie, breech presentation of the first twin.

The very first eye-contact and intensive physical contact with both my twins: Approx. 6 to 7 hours after the operation.

The following complications occurred with breastfeeding after the second Caesarean: Stress, extreme puerperal depression: I expressed milk (2 months).

I would have preferred natural (vaginal) births: Yes.

I was afraid of pain during birth/of perineal trauma: No.

I was afraid of a possible Caesarean section with the second birth: Yes.

I miss having a natural birth experience: Yes.

I feel inferior due to having missed out on the experience of birth: Yes.

I experienced the Caesarean sections as traumatic: Not the first but the second.

The Caesarean section was the ideal way of giving birth as far as I am concerned: No.

Due to the following the rate of Caesareans is rising: Children grow faster than they used to and are therefore larger, nature cannot keep up. It is a kind of "safer birth" – at least for the child!

My fundamental attitude on the topic "Caesarean": If it is important for mother and child (or the mother is afraid) then it is good. For the sake of convenience or just out of laziness I personally entertain some doubt.

My Caesarean scar (length approx. 18 cm):

It makes my stomach bulge out. This bothers me a lot. Seen from the front and from the left to the right the appendix scar fades into the Caesarean scar and the hernia. After the first Caesarean I had a totally flat stomach. With the second Caesarean the tissue was displaced and my stomach was blue for about a month.

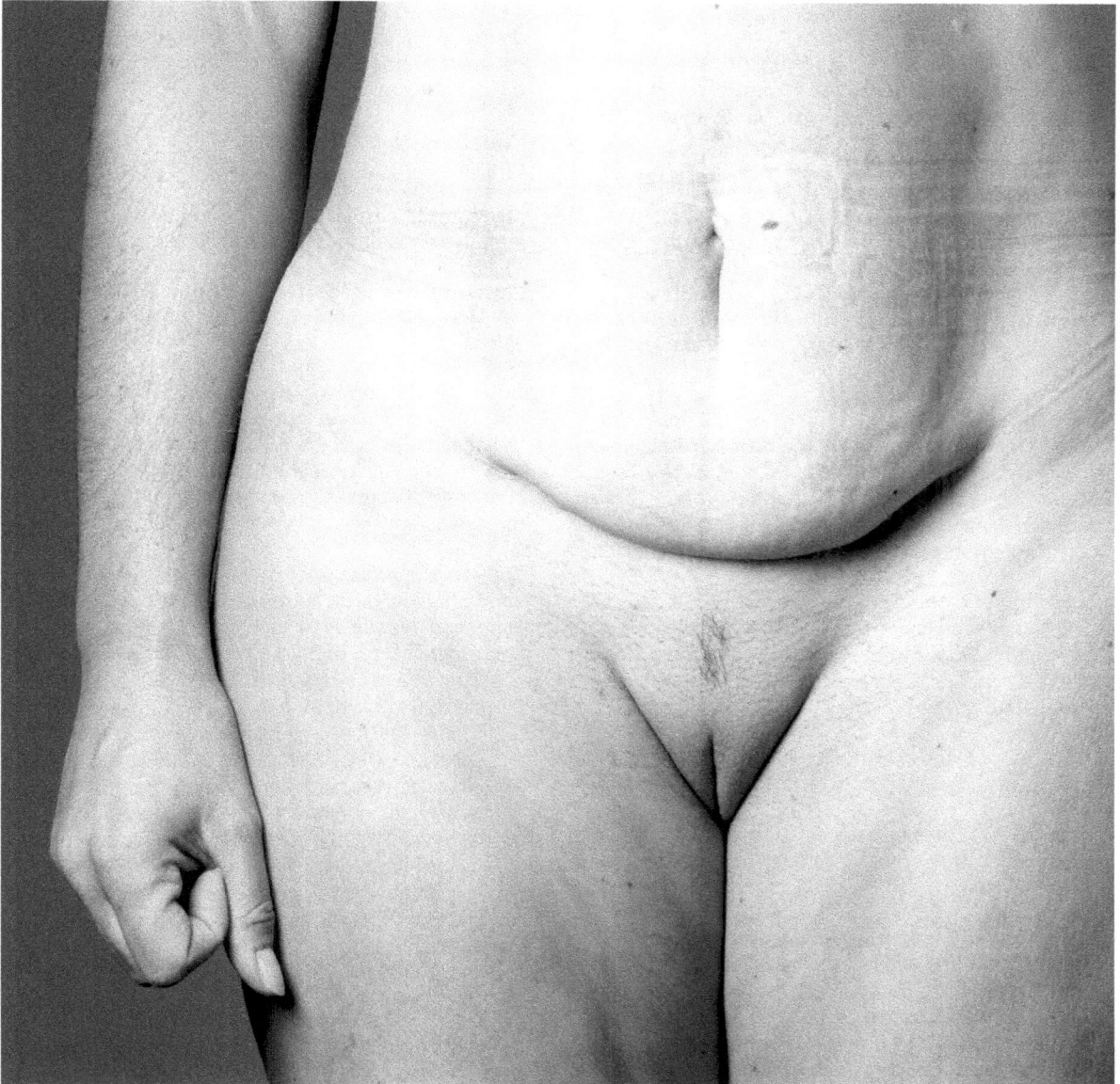

[T062]   I find an elective Caesarean section difficult to understand:

But what happens when the obstetrician does not trust himself to do it because of lack of experience?!?

Occupation: Registered physiotherapist.

When I hear the word "Caesarean section" the following words come to mind spontaneously: Immobile, pain, hospitalisation, complicated care for the child, saving mother and/or child.

The birth of my first child (vaginal delivery): 9.20 p.m. beautiful, premature rupture of membranes, was fit after birth (shower, midnight snack), went home the following morning.

The birth of my second child (vaginal delivery): 10.25 p.m. see above, rupture of membranes 3 weeks before term.

The birth of my third child (first section): Contractions: No. Head circumference 33.5 cm, height 48 cm, weight 2416 g, duration of pregnancy: 37 weeks. Section due to placenta praevia: Could prepare, additional complication – onset of preeclampsia. Very bad thrombocyte readings – massive bleeding.

The following complications occurred with the first Caesarean section: I did not have enough thrombocytes due to preeclampsia – disturbed blood clotting – post-operative bleeding – reoperated under general anaesthesia.

The first intensive physical contact with my third child: Approx. 30 minutes after the operation.

I was able to breastfeed without difficulty after the first Caesarean: I breastfed for more than a year.

The birth of my fourth child (second section): Contractions: No. Head circumference 34.6 cm, height 51 cm, weight 2540 g, duration of pregnancy: 34 weeks +5 days. Acute, because of decreasing thrombocyte readings – no time to prepare, also too early for the child (4 weeks before term) – 3 days neonatal ward.

The indication for my second section: HELLP syndrome, pathological Doppler ultrasound, massive decrease in mother's thrombocytes due to preeclampsia: danger of blood clotting disorder.

The first intensive physical contact with my fourth child: Approx. 43 hours after the operation.

My fourth child had serious health problems: Adaptive difficulties, breathing problems.

I was able to breastfeed without difficulty after the second Caesarean: I breastfed for more than 2 years.

I ascribe the following peculiarities of my fourth child to the Caesarean birth: To a lesser extent to the section than to the consequences of sudden surgery (= transfer to neonatal ward): extreme need for cuddling, difficulties parting, difficulties with transitions (sleeping – being awake).

Due to the following the rate of Caesareans is rising: Fear of birth, fear of complications during birth, increased readiness to sue when complications occur: surgeons cut earlier, it is said to be safer. Young obstetricians are not trained in certain situations occurring during birth, as part of their training anymore [...]: Things that used to be routine are, therefore, really getting riskier. [...] Nothing is left to chance with an only child planned very late and every imaginable risk is eliminated. Nobody is informed about the risks of the section. The Caesarean section is presented as a painless alternative to the painful birth – which is not true! You might (perhaps) not have labour pains before, but therefore you are immobile for quite a while afterwards, cannot care for your child on your own, have to stay in hospital for a week, have pain when getting up, laughing, ...

My Caesarean scar (length approx. 14 cm):

When the children play around on my tummy I sometimes feel a stabbing
pain. But it is getting less. My Caesarean scar is inconspicuous. Not
so the appendix scar which I have had since I was 11.

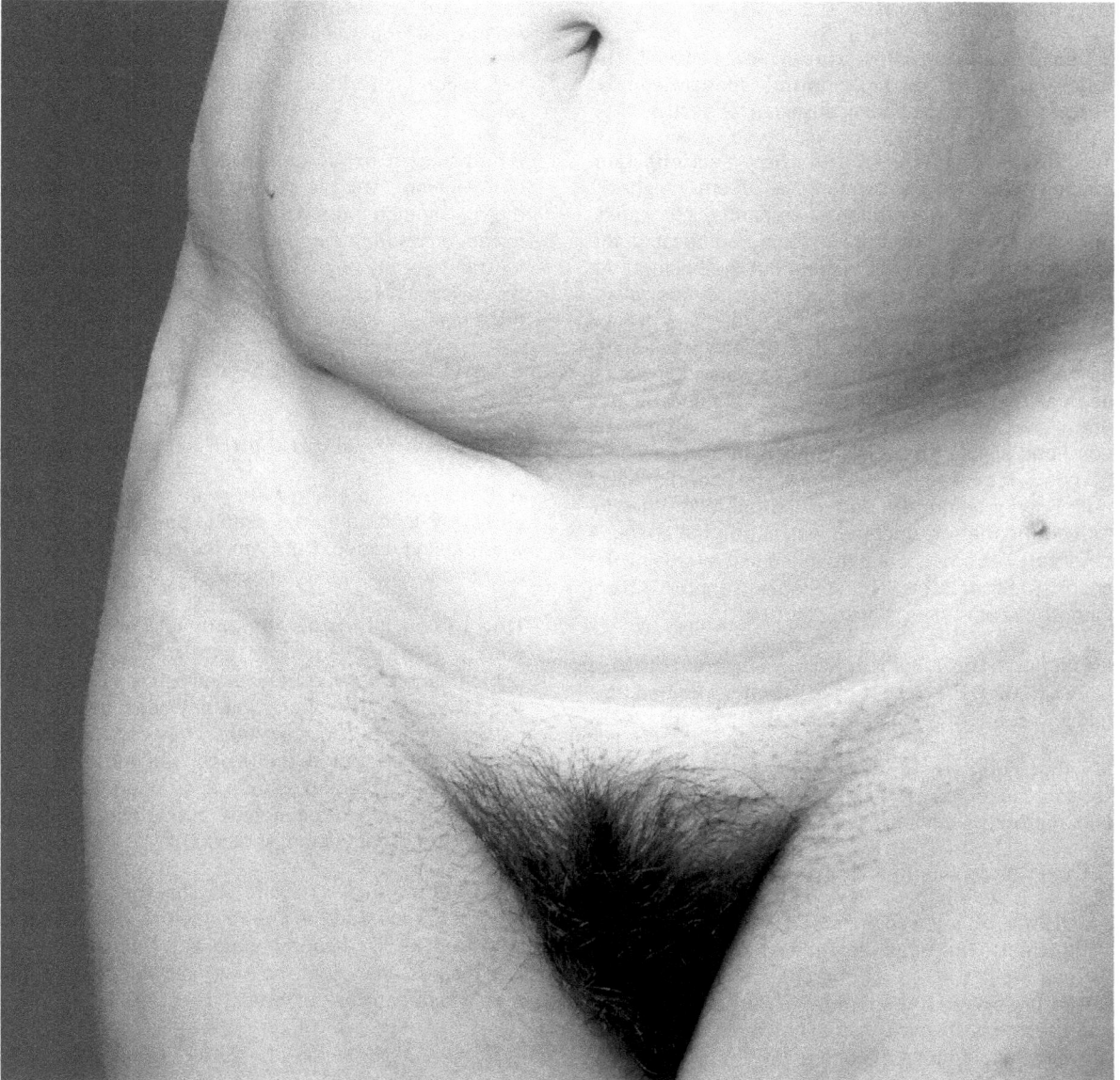

[T113]   The indication for both my sections:

A cerebral haemorrhage at the age of 17. As this haemorrhage healed by itself and was not operated on, the danger of complications during a spontaneous birth would have been too high. I was not allowed to have pushing contractions.

Occupation: Office worker.

When I hear the word "Caesarean section" the following words come to mind spontaneously: Surgery, pain, helplessness, anxieties, anaesthesia.

The birth of my first child (first section): Contractions: No. Head circumference 37 cm, height 51 cm, weight 4130 g, duration of pregnancy: 39 weeks. Anxiety during the anaesthesia (epidural) because the obstetrician was not able to carry out the epidural. After the third or fourth try another physician was called. He was able to administer the epidural. I was a total wreck and the obstetrician asked me what was wrong, as if nothing had happened. I was very afraid of lasting damage (paralysis amongst others). My husband was not allowed to be with me. After the Caesarean section I had signs of paralysis in my right foot for about 36 hours. It improved the next day. The operation went well. Shortly before the end of the operation they informed me that my daughter was cut on the cheek. A physician was present and attended to it by glueing the cheek. The scar is 2 to 3 mm broad and approx. 3.5 cm long. The scar is still visible today.

I did not suffer from depression after the first Caesarean: But I did not have anyone, who had also had a Caesarean section, to talk to.

My first child was injured through the Caesarean section: Cut on the left cheek (approx. 2 to 3 mm broad and approx. 3.5 cm long; see page 17).

My first child has health problems now: Eczema.

The birth of my second child (second section): Contractions: No. Head circumference 36 cm, height 54 cm, weight 4318 g, duration of pregnancy: 39 weeks. I was already prepared for a Caesarean section. The anaesthesia went well but I had massive problems with circulation during the operation.

My second child was injured through the Caesarean section: Minute scratch on the ear.

My second child has health problems now: Eczema.

I had health problems after my second Caesarean section: After the second Caesarean I always felt a dragging pain around the scar and had no feeling in my abdomen for a long time, which was a big problem for me. I got my physical well-being back after having the meridians activated (Chinese massage). Now I feel great again.

I would have preferred natural (vaginal) births: Yes.

I miss having a natural birth experience: Yes.

A Caesarean birth possibly has effects on the child: My children always need to be close to me also when falling asleep. But I am not sure if this can be ascribed to the Caesarean birth.

Due to the following the rate of Caesareans is rising: There is too much uncertainty about what could happen, caused by gynaecologists as well as by acquaintances. There are too many negative influences from all sides (TV, newspaper, friends, physicians). Women should get to hear and see more positive things. The Caesarean section is an operation (which should not be underestimated), but no one points out the risks (e.g. cuts amongst others).

My fundamental attitude on the topic "Caesarean": It is good that the possibility exists. But it should only be done if it is appropriate. But I am very happy that the possibility exists so that I was able to have children without any risk to myself.

My Caesarean scars (length approx. 10 cm):

I was aware of my Caesarean scar in the following way: A strong dragging pain upwards and downwards, as if one wants to pull the abdomen apart. Since my treatment a few months ago (activating meridians) I have no problems anymore. I used to massage my Caesarean scar softly.

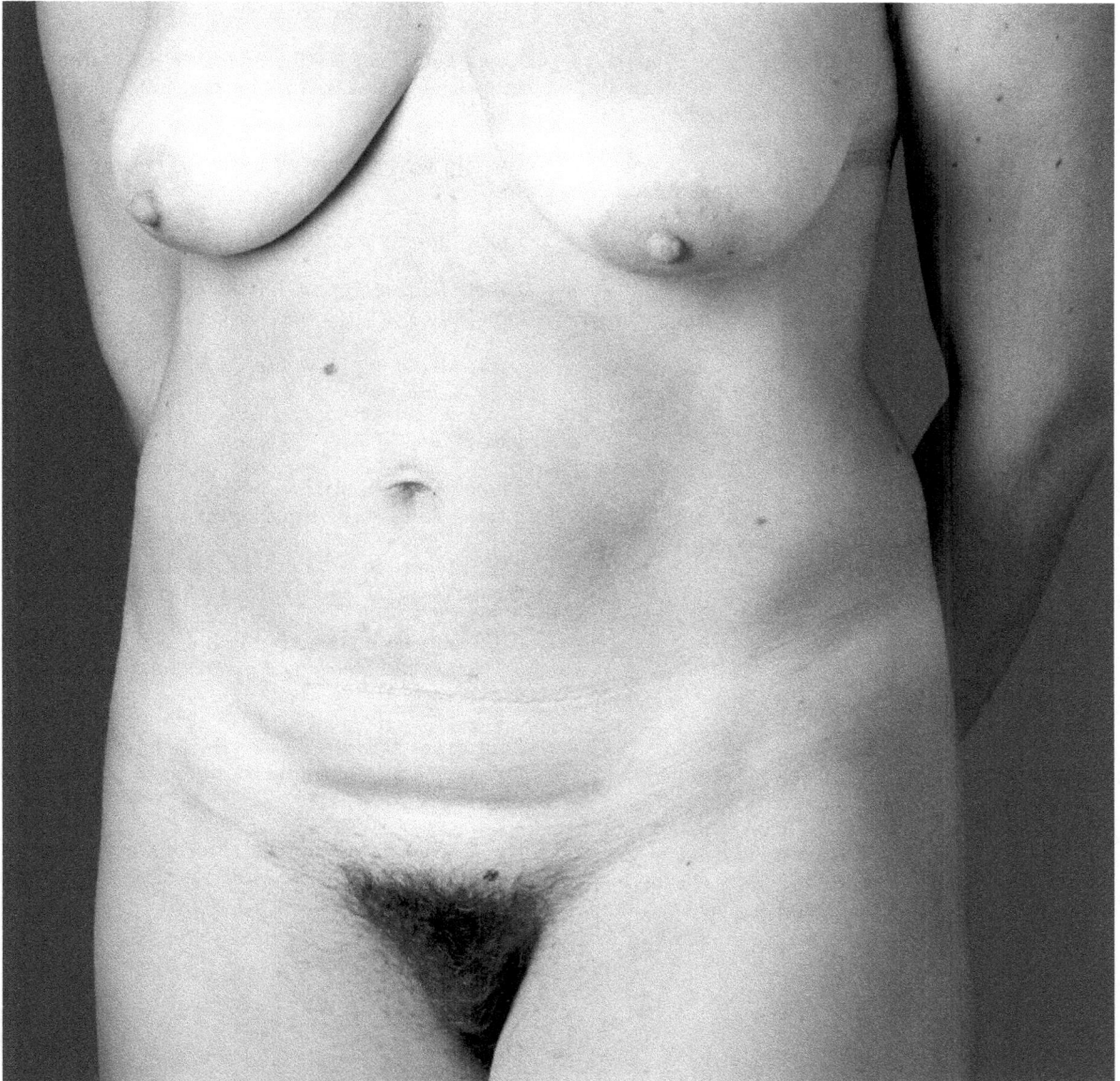

If there is no other possibility then "it" should be done
– but not because it is fashionable.

Occupation: Agriculturist.

When I hear the word "Caesarean section" the following words come to mind spontaneously: Failure, my poor child, what a beginning to life, why can I not give birth, have I done something wrong.

I dealt with Caesareans intensively prior to my first Caesarean birth: No.

The birth of my first child (first section): Induced labour: Approx. 15 hours. Head circumference 40 cm, height 49 cm, weight 3490 g, duration of pregnancy n.s. My child was clinically dead (4 minutes).

The indication for my first section: My child's oxygen deficiency.

The first Caesarean proceeded without complications: Yes.

I had problems breastfeeding after the first Caesarean: I only saw my child 5 days later.

The first Caesarean interfered with the mother-child bonding: The children have got no basic trust.

My first child had serious health problems: Bronchitis, allergies.

My first child has health problems now: No.

The birth of my second child (second section): Induced labour: Approx. 1 hour. Head circumference 37 cm, height 54 cm, weight 4080 g, duration of pregnancy: 41 weeks. I have the feeling that the Caesarean was planned from the beginning.

The indication for my second section: n.s.

I was able to breastfeed without difficulty after the second Caesarean: I breastfed for more than 1 year.

I would have preferred natural (vaginal) births: Yes.

I miss having a natural birth experience: Yes.

I feel inferior due to having missed out on the experience of birth: Yes.

I was afraid of a possible Caesarean section: No.

I experienced both Caesarean sections as traumatic: Yes.

The Caesarean births give me the feeling of not having done everything for my children: Yes.

The Caesarean section was the ideal way of giving birth as far as I am concerned: No.

A Caesarean birth possibly has negative effects on the child: It feels as if my children take longer to trust someone.

I find that Caesarean section is trivialised and minimised by the media (newspaper, magazines, television, ...): Yes.

Due to the following the rate of Caesareans is rising: People think the birth can take place along with other appointments. Fear of pain.

My Caesarean scar (length approx. 18 cm):

The wound only healed after 3 months. I feel my Caesarean scar with weather changes.
I find my Caesarean scar ugly. It is not easy for me to touch my Caesarean scar.

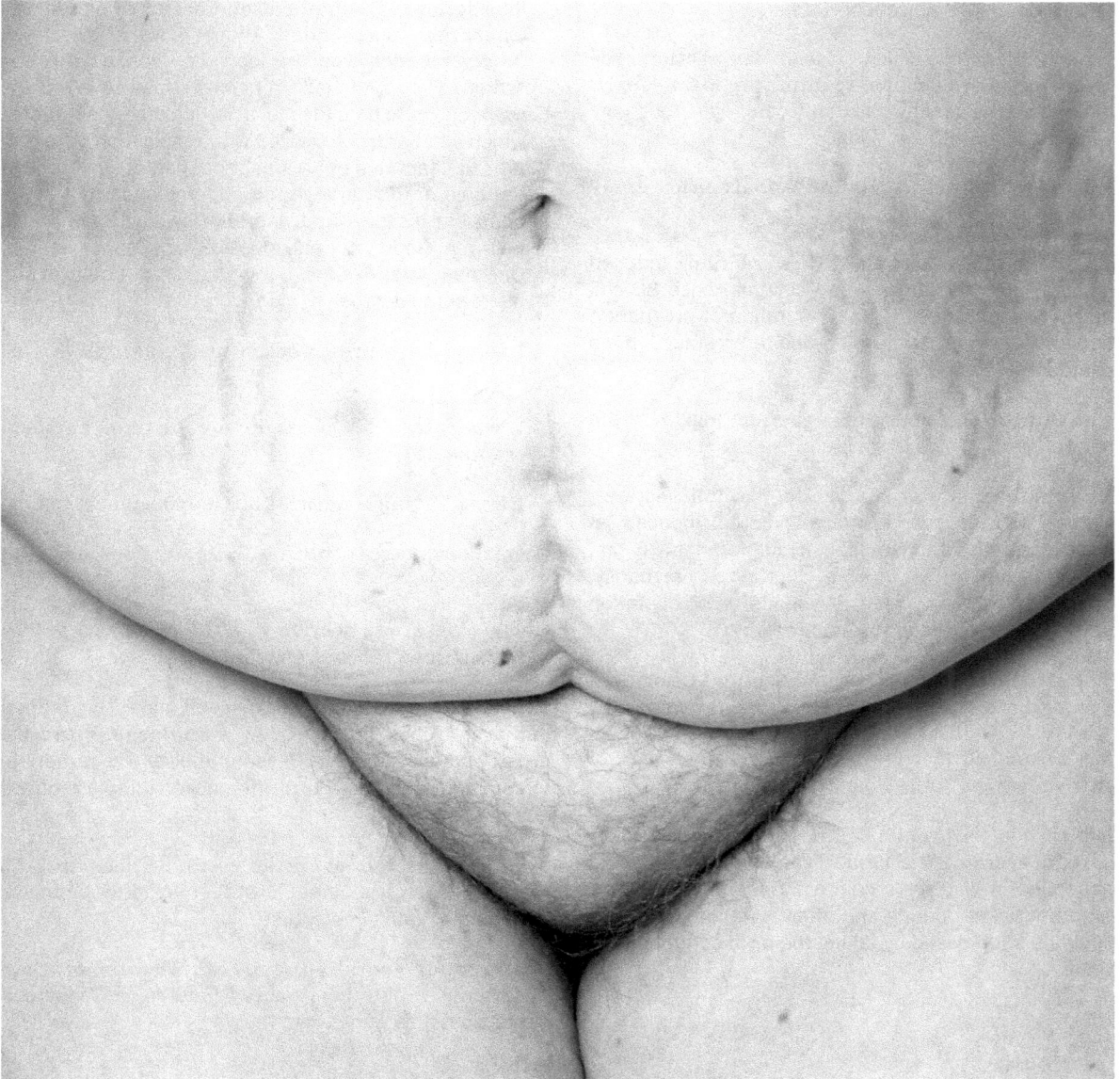

[T068] I have given birth to two children and had a Caesarean section twice:

A third laparotomy was done when my uterus had to be removed because of extensive adhesions.

Occupation: Middle school teacher.

When I hear the word "Caesarean section" the following words come to mind spontaneously: Major surgery, healthy children, scars, pain, long convalescence.

I dealt with Caesareans intensively prior to my first Caesarean birth: No.

The birth of my first child (first section): Induced labour: Approx. 5 hours. Head circumference 36 cm, height 54 cm, weight 3550 g, duration of pregnancy: approx. 42 weeks. 14 days beyond term, induction, no dilatation of the cervix.

The indication for my first section: Rigidity of the cervix, the child's heart tones.

The birth of my second child (second section): Natural contractions: Approx. 12 hours. Induced labour: Approx. 5 hours. Head circumference 36 cm, height 52 cm, weight 3550 g, duration of pregnancy: approx. 43 weeks. 3 weeks beyond term, no dilatation of the cervix despite strong contractions.

The indication for my second section: Being overdue, rigidity of the cervix, the child's heart tones.

My second child was injured through the Caesarean section: Little wound on the cheek.

I had health problems after the second Caesarean section: The broad ligament grew onto the abdominal wall: Severe pain every month for approx. 14 days (before, during and after ovulation). The pain could be suppressed by taking the birth control pill for years.

The following complications occurred when my Caesarean scar healed: After removal of the uterus (through the scar from the second section) a nerve was "stitched" in. "Stitched" in nerves cause severe pains (happens from time to time, also with other operations) which can hardly be treated with medication. After approx. 4 years this nerve finally calmed down. Through the pain of the nerve in the abdominal cavity I developed bad posture and, thereby, low-back pain, neck pain etc. Sport was only possible to a minor degree. Only now, after 4 years (!) the state of my health is stable to some degree.

I would have preferred natural (vaginal) births: Yes.

I was afraid of pain during birth/of perineal trauma: No.

I miss having a natural birth experience: Yes.

I experienced both Caesarean sections as traumatic: Yes.

The Caesarean section was the ideal way of giving birth as far as I am concerned: No.

My Caesarean births are seen as fully-fledged births by my family, friends and acquaintances: Yes and no. In 1981 a Caesarean birth was rather uncommon, therefore I was often asked if I had requested it!

Due to the following the rate of Caesareans is rising: Fear of perineal laceration, bladder problems and pain during intercourse.

My fundamental attitude on the topic "Caesarean": If birth can proceed naturally a Caesarean should not be done.

My Caesarean scars (length approx. 15 cm):

My scars are – according to my current gynaecologist – set 5 cm too high. Both Caesarean sections were performed by a surgeon who rarely operated and therefore lacked experience.

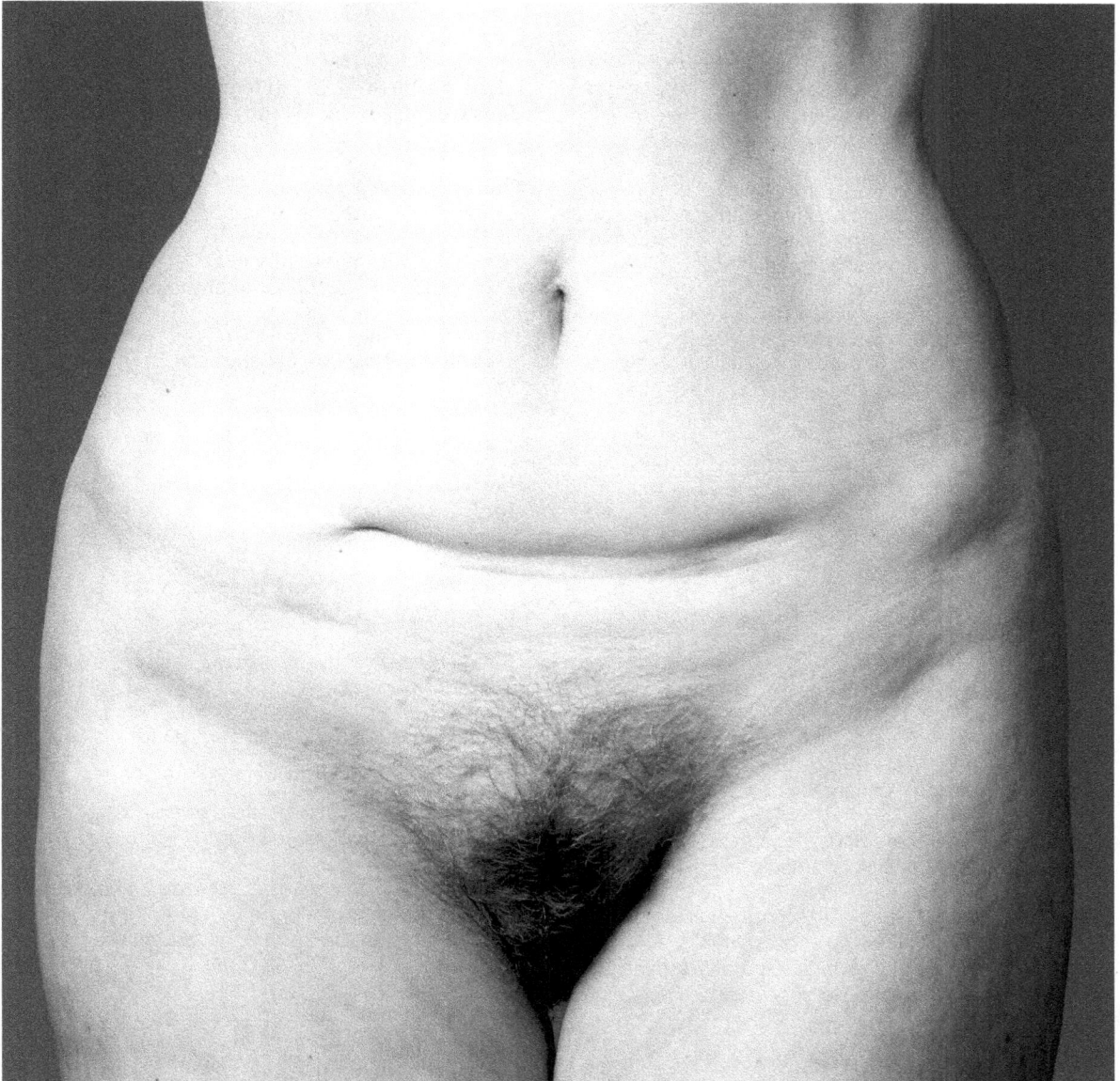

[T027] After the death of my second child a gynaecologist told me:

"You will never have a child!"

Occupation: Civil servant

When I hear the word "Caesarean section" the following words come to mind spontaneously: High-risk delivery, high-risk pregnancy – possible miscarriage, possible difficulties breastfeeding, pain, prettier children.

The birth of my first child (vaginal delivery): Miscarriage in the 26th week of pregnancy. Intrauterine growth impairment of the child: died in womb.

The birth of my second child (first section): Contractions: No. Head circumference n.s., height 30 cm, weight 570 g, duration of pregnancy: 26 weeks. Again 26th week of pregnancy (5 weeks earlier in hospital for monitoring), child died 13 days after birth.

The indication for my first section: Intrauterine growth impairment of the child.

I wanted to breastfeed after birth: Neonatal ward – child died of heart failure.

The very first eye-contact with my second child: Approx. 24 hours after the operation.

The first intensive physical contact with my second child: N.s.

I suffered from depression after the first Caesarean: But only after my daughter's death.

My second child had health problems: Immature lungs, was on 8 of the 10 life support machines.

The birth of my third child (second section): Contractions: No. Height 49 cm, weight 3160 g, duration of pregnancy: 37 weeks. A picture-perfect pregnancy thanks to my homoeopath. Delivery in the 37th week of pregnancy – planned.

The indication for my second section: High-risk pregnancy due to history.

I had problems breastfeeding after the second Caesarean section: My son rejected the breast. I did not breastfeed.

The very first eye-contact with my third child: Approx. 1 hour after the operation.

The first intensive physical contact with my third child: Approx. 1 hour after the operation.

The second Caesarean interfered with the mother-child bonding: No, not anymore.

My third child had serious health problems: Pollen allergy. Healed by injections (3 ½ years).

I ascribe the following peculiarities of my third child to the Caesarean birth: Above average intelligence, however minimalist, likes staying at home.

I would have preferred natural (vaginal) births: Yes.

I was afraid of pain during birth/of perineal trauma: No.

I experienced both Caesarean sections as traumatic: No.

The Caesarean was the ideal way of giving birth as far as I am concerned: No.

Due to the following the rate of Caesareans is rising: Because women are different. Maybe too narrow, and they do not know enough about the risks of surgery.

My fundamental attitude on the topic "Caesarean": Decide for the benefit of the mother and despite all watch the child's health.

My Caesarean scars (length approx. 18 cm):

The surgeon was very careful. The smaller scar is from my daughter.
Despite the rush they did not cut from the navel to the pubic hair. The
second scar is a lot larger. But cut with accuracy and skill.

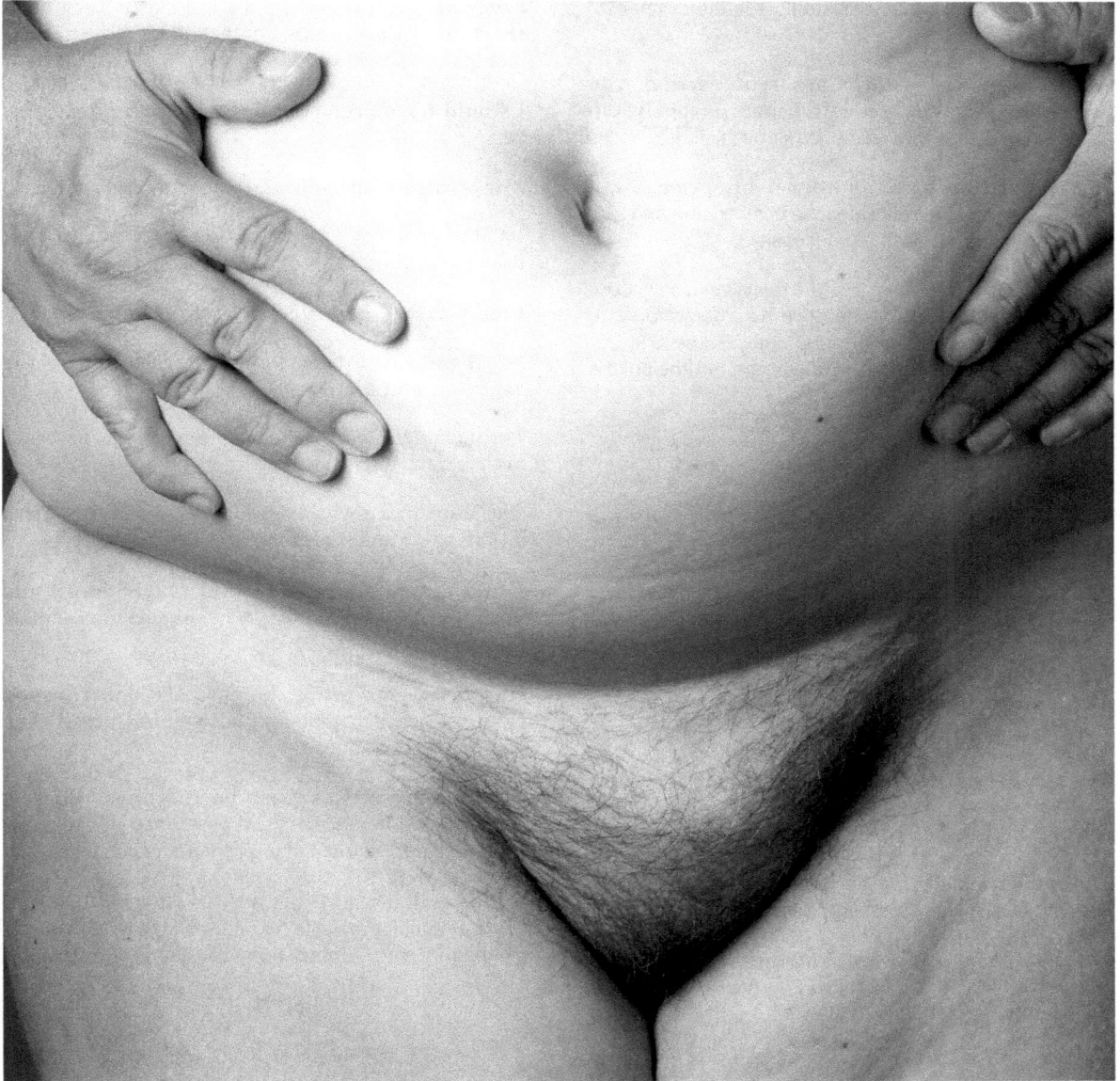

Back then a Caesarean was an absolute exception
there. The surgeon had studied in the USA.

Occupation: Personal assistant, recruiter, import/export.

When I hear the word "Caesarean section" the following words come to mind spontaneously: Unnatural birth, missing experience of birth.

I dealt with Caesareans intensively prior to my first Caesarean birth: Because obstetrician and surgeon predicted the possible necessity.

The birth of my first child (first section): Contractions: No. Head circumference n.s., height 53 cm, weight 3030 g, duration of pregnancy: 38 weeks. Difficult decision in favour of a Caesarean, but the child's health has top priority!

The indication for my first section: Very strong abdominal muscles, the baby could not drop.

The very first eye-contact with my first child: Approx. 1 hour after the operation.

The first intensive physical contact with my first child: Approx. 2 hours after the operation.

I was able to breastfeed without difficulty after the first Caesarean: I breastfed for a couple of months.

The birth of my second child (second section): Contractions: No. Height 50 cm, weight 3490 g, duration of pregnancy: 38 weeks. Caesarean accepted.

The indication for my second section: Very strong abdominal muscles – see first Caesarean.

The very first eye-contact and intensive physical contact with my second child: Approx. 1 hour after the operation.

I was able to breastfeed without difficulty after the second Caesarean: I breastfed for more than six months.

I would have preferred natural (vaginal) births: Yes.

I was afraid of pain during birth/of perineal trauma: No.

I was afraid of a possible Caesarean section: No.

I miss having a natural birth experience: Yes.

I feel inferior due to having missed out on the experience of birth: No.

I experienced both Caesarean sections as traumatic: No.

The Caesarean was the ideal way of giving birth as far as I am concerned: No.

I find that Caesarean section is trivialised and minimised by the media (newspaper, magazines, television, ...): Yes.

Due to the following the rate of Caesareans is rising: Exact scheduling is possible for obstetrician and mother, fear of pain.

My fundamental attitude on the topic "Caesarean": Should actually only be performed in situations that are life-threatening for mother or child.

Additional notes: I was a gymnast from 12 to 20 years of age. From 20 to 26 years of age I did rhythmic gymnastics, furthermore horseback riding and skiing.

My Caesarean scar (length approx. 13 cm):

The scar of the second Caesarean became infected. It was very easy
for me to accept my scar as it is well covered by pubic hair.

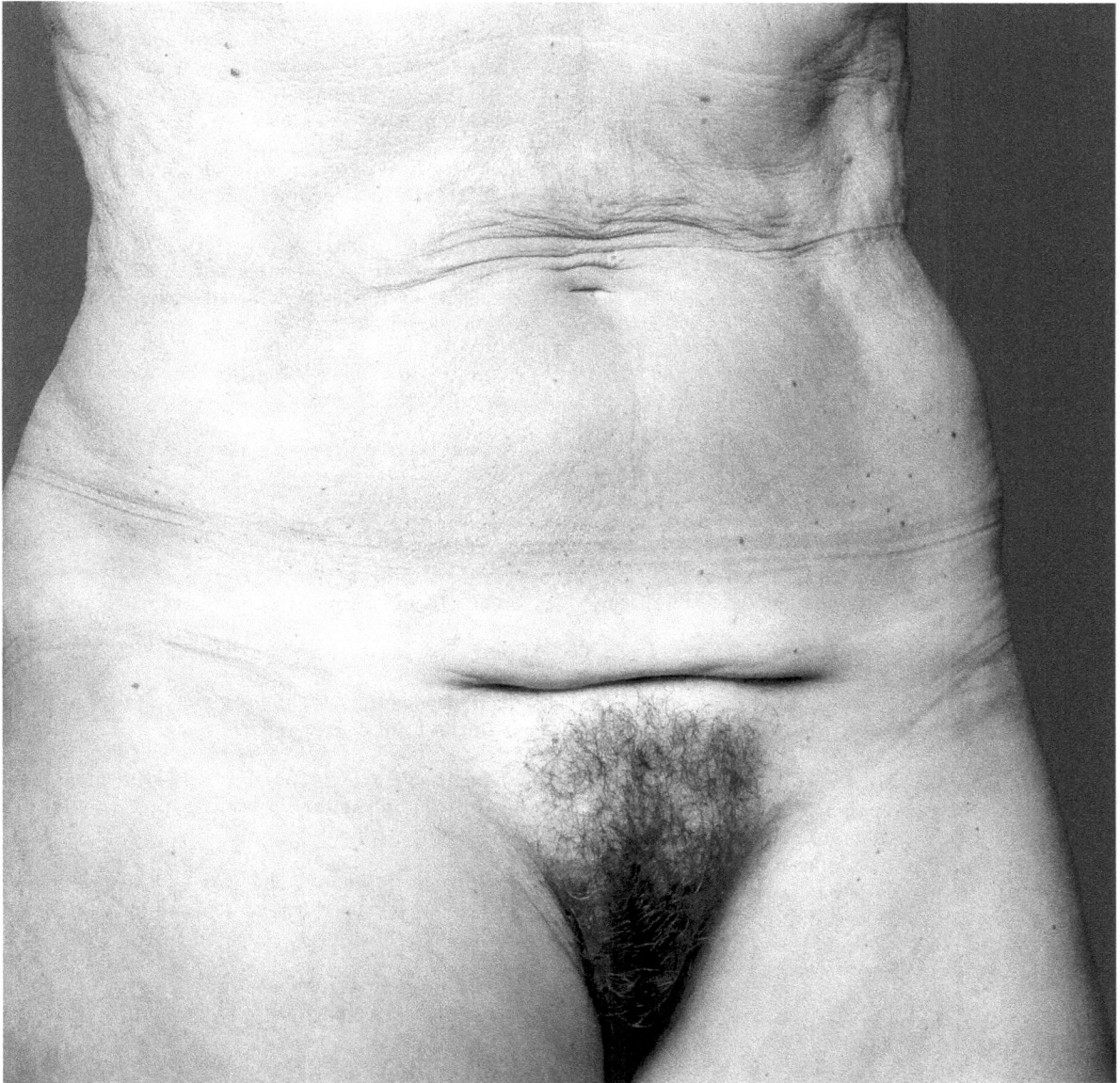

My children are 42 and 40 years old – everything happened a very long time ago. Back then there was not a lot of education, especially in my case. The children were born in Athens, communication with the physician was in English, there was no contact with the midwife. I have forgotten and also repressed a lot, therefore it is difficult for me to fill in the questionnaire properly.

Occupation: Retired.

When I hear the word "Caesarean section" the following words come to mind spontaneously: n.s.

I dealt with Caesareans intensively prior to my first Caesarean birth: No.

The birth of my first child (first section): Natural contractions: Approx. 6 to 7 hours. Head circumference n.s., height 52 cm, weight 4200 g, duration of pregnancy: 40 weeks. "Birthday" exactly on the calculated day. Contractions came and went, after approx. 6 hours the Caesarean had to be done, birth canal would not open.

The indication for my first section: n.s.

The very first eye-contact and intensive physical contact with my first child: ?

I had problems breastfeeding after the first Caesarean: I had a fever, breastfeeding was discontinued.

The first Caesarean interfered with the mother-child bonding: I was so weak after the operation that I could not enjoy the physical contact.

The birth of my second child (second section): Contractions: No. Head circumference n.s., height 50 cm, weight 3800 g, duration of pregnancy: 38 weeks. Back then (1966) they said "once a Caesarean, always a Caesarean". It was performed two weeks before the calculated time. I had to wait in a room adjoining the operating theatre for one hour. Then I was in the operating theatre for a very long time (don't know why).

The indication for my second section: Once a Caesarean, always a Caesarean.

The following complications occurred during the second Caesarean: I was in the operating theatre for a very long time, I never found out why. The lower part of the "Caesarean section" was left open, the cannula was only removed days later.

The very first eye-contact and intensive physical contact with my second child: ?

The second Caesarean interfered with the mother-child bonding: It is not a real experience of birth. After surgery (under general anaesthetic) it takes a while to be fully there.

I wanted to breastfeed after the second Caesarean birth: No.

I would have preferred natural (vaginal) births: Yes.

I was afraid of pain during birth/of perineal trauma: n.s.

I was afraid of a possible Caesarean section: n.s.

I miss having a natural birth experience: n.s.

The Caesarean was the ideal way of giving birth as far as I am concerned: No.

I find that Caesarean section is trivialised and minimised by the media (newspaper, magazines, television, ...): Yes.

Due to the following the rate of Caesareans is rising: Free of pain, quick, scar hardly visible (can supposedly also be removed by laser).

My fundamental attitude on the topic "Caesarean": It should be an emergency solution.

My Caesarean scar (length approx. 15 cm):

My Caesarean scar did not heal trouble-free because one part was left open and healed very slowly. I had to wear a surgical corset. At my age the appearance of the scar is not important anymore but it used to bother me in the past. I had complexes because the scar was so noticeable. I only wore high-cut bikini bottoms.

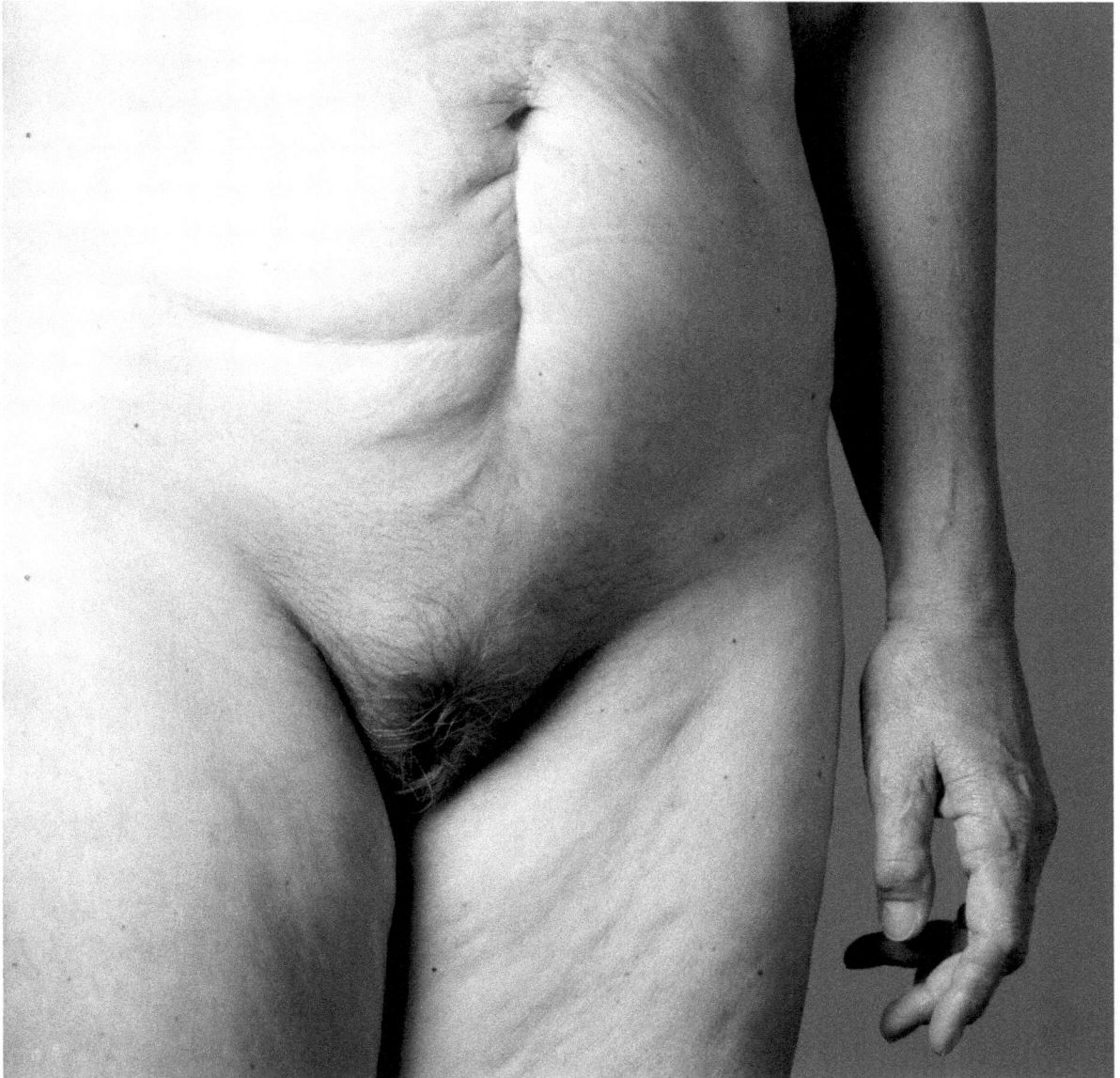

Caesarean mothers with two sections

Caesarean mothers with three sections

[T010]   The third section had the following indication:

Two previous Caesareans.

Occupation: Employee. At present: maternity leave.

When I hear the word "Caesarean section" the following words come to mind spontaneously: Pain, fear, emergency solution, complications.

The birth of my first child (first section): Natural contractions: Approx. 10 hours. Head circumference 34 cm, height 53 cm, weight 2820 g, duration of pregnancy: 36 weeks +6 days. Did unfortunately not deal with the topic of the "section", was very surprising for us.

The indication for my first section: Malpresentation of the child (brow presentation), fever, foetal tachycardia.

The birth of my second child (second section): Natural contractions: Approx. 10 hours. Head circumference 36 cm, height 54 cm, weight 3800 g, duration of pregnancy: 38 weeks +6 days. It was a little more relaxed as I had an epidural during the entire birth. Despite this, it was again very unexpected.

The indication for my second section: Malposition of the child, uterine atony.

The birth of my third child (third section): Contractions: No. Head circumference 36 cm, height 55 cm, weight 3480 g, duration of pregnancy: 38 weeks +1 day.

The third Caesarean section was: Planned.

The third Caesarean section was: Not an emergency section nor an elective section.

The decision in favour of the third Caesarean: Was made by the physician in the end.

The third Caesarean proceeded without complications: Yes.

The very first eye-contact and intensive physical contact with my third child: During the operation.

The Caesarean interfered with the mother-child bonding: No.

I was afraid of pain during birth or of perineal trauma: No.

I was afraid of a possible third Caesarean section: Yes.

Additional notes: Time goes by way too fast and nine months are over so quickly. I also lost 13 kilos. Would be ready for a photo shoot now. ☺ I can only add to the book that this was the "most beautiful Caesarean" I have ever had. I was very nervous and could not sleep all night but everything went well. The whole operation was really relaxed. Five hours later they already removed the needle from my hand and I did not need any painkillers. I don't know why! Maybe because I had the operation without long labour and I had rested before. The following days were also great! I was able to breastfeed my child without difficulty and also had little pain when getting up and walking. I was allowed to leave the hospital on the fifth day. Thank God, cause I am not a fan of such institutions. [...] If I had had the opportunity to deliver normally despite two Caesareans, I would have done it. Unfortunately, obstetricians are not enthusiastic about that. I am curious about the statements of the women who have had four Caesareans. You never know!!! Our home is quite big.

My Caesarean scar (length approx. 15 cm):

Up to this moment I have not had a single problem with the scar. As my varicose vein was not allowed to be injured, it is two centimetres longer than the two previous ones (the old scars are 13 cm and the new one is 15 cm).

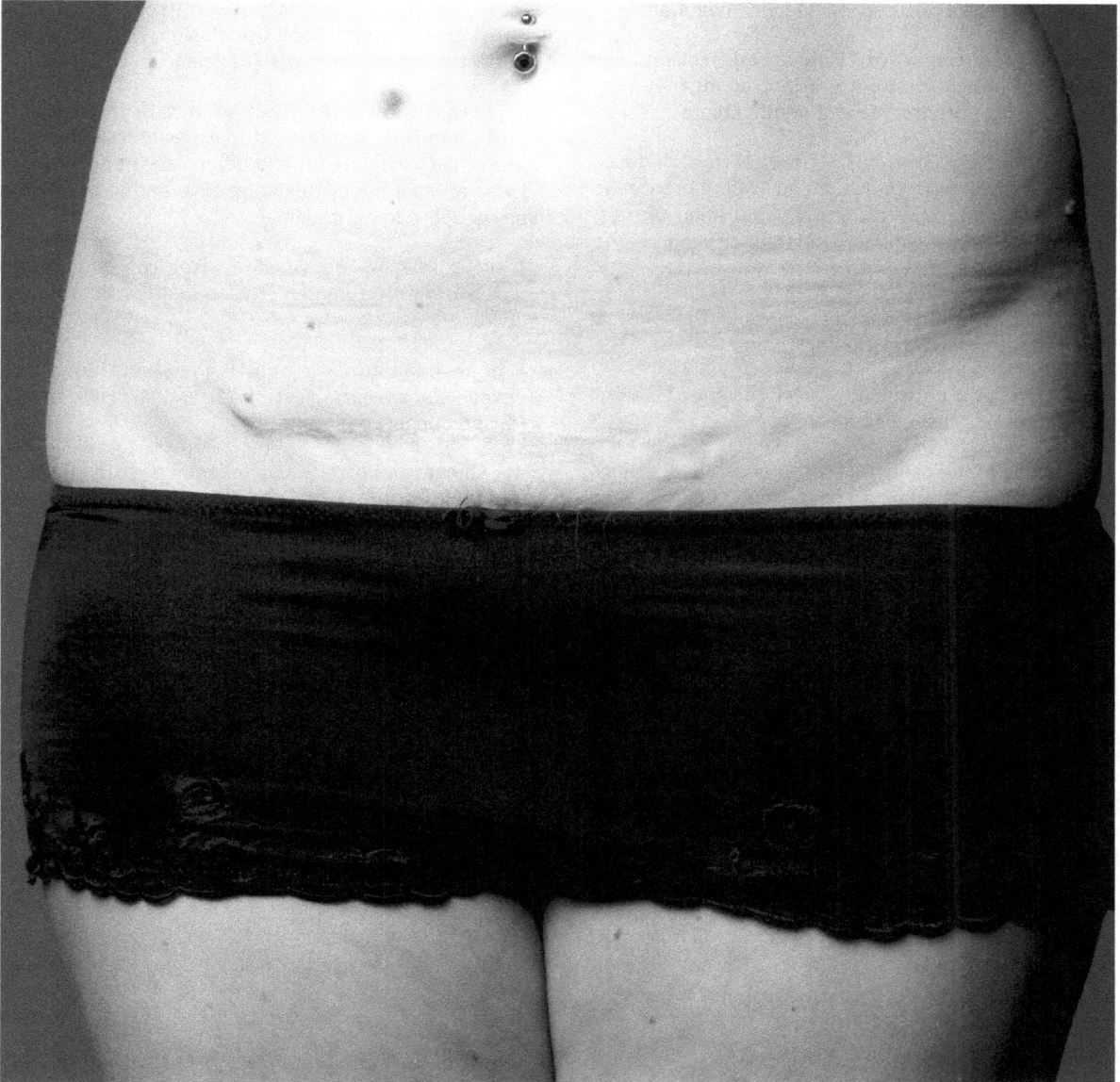

Caesarean mothers with three sections

[T074] I thought I was going to die of pain:

> I became apathetic in the car, just wanted to be in hospital [...]. When I arrived in the maternity room there were no more heart tones, my child had turned completely. That sounds relatively obvious, but everybody was totally confused at first, there was nothing visible on the ultrasound (due to all the blood from the rupture – the old Caesarean scar had opened up). [...] A physician then told me that my daughter had died.

Occupation: Grammar school teacher, historian.

When I hear the word "Caesarean section" the following words come to mind spontaneously: Surgery, pain, surprise, life and death, failure.

The birth of my first child (first section): Induced labour: Approx. 30 minutes. Head circumference 35 cm, height 50 cm, weight 2950 g, duration of pregnancy: 42 weeks. Secondary emergency section after induction.

The indication for my first section: Pathological CTG after induction with prostaglandin.

I suffered from depression after the first Caesarean: Deep, long-lasting sadness (approx. 1 year).

The birth of my second child (second section): Induced labour: Approx. 4 hours. Head circumference 34.5 cm, height 49 cm, weight 3100 g, duration of pregnancy: 42 weeks. Secondary emergency section after induction.

The indication for my second section: Pathological CTG after induction with oxytocin.

I suffered from depression after the second Caesarean: Deep, long-lasting sadness (approx. 1 ½ years).

The birth of my third child (third section): Natural contractions: Approx. 5 hours until uterine rupture, another 2 hours until section. Head circumference 35 cm, height 50 cm, weight 3400 g, duration of pregnancy: 42 weeks. Emergency section after uterine rupture.

The indication for my third section: Uterine rupture.

The following complications occurred during the third Caesarean: Blood transfusion. Stillbirth of my daughter (caused by oxygen deficiency).

The third Caesarean interfered with the mother-child bonding: It is difficult to explain this with a still-born child. Compared to the other Caesarean sections I was at least happy to still be alive and to be able to say goodbye to my daughter.

I suffered from depression after the third Caesarean: Post-traumatic problems after death of a child.

I have been having health problems since my three Caesarean sections: Psychological strain. Raised danger of rupture.

My Caesarean births are not seen as fully-fledged births by my family, friends and acquaintances: Not being able to join conversations, it is seen as more of an illness.

A Caesarean birth possibly has negative effects on the child: Bonding problems, anxiety, agitated.

Due to the following the rate of Caesareans is rising: Reputed to be an "easy" birth, following pregnancies often again Caesarean, scheduling, regarding invoicing the hospital is better off.

My fundamental attitude on the topic "Caesarean": Anger about trivialisation and quick decision in favour of the Caesarean section, but due to stillbirth also knowledgeable about lifesaving function of Caesareans.

My Caesarean scar (length approx. 15 cm):

I hardly feel my Caesarean scar, sometimes a dragging pain. I am quite happy that at least the physical scar healed well. Although it is a contradiction to the deep mental scar. The fact that such a beautifully healed scar tears, makes me feel as if I've been cheated. Statistically seen the rupture is such a rare complication – I never thought that it would hit me.

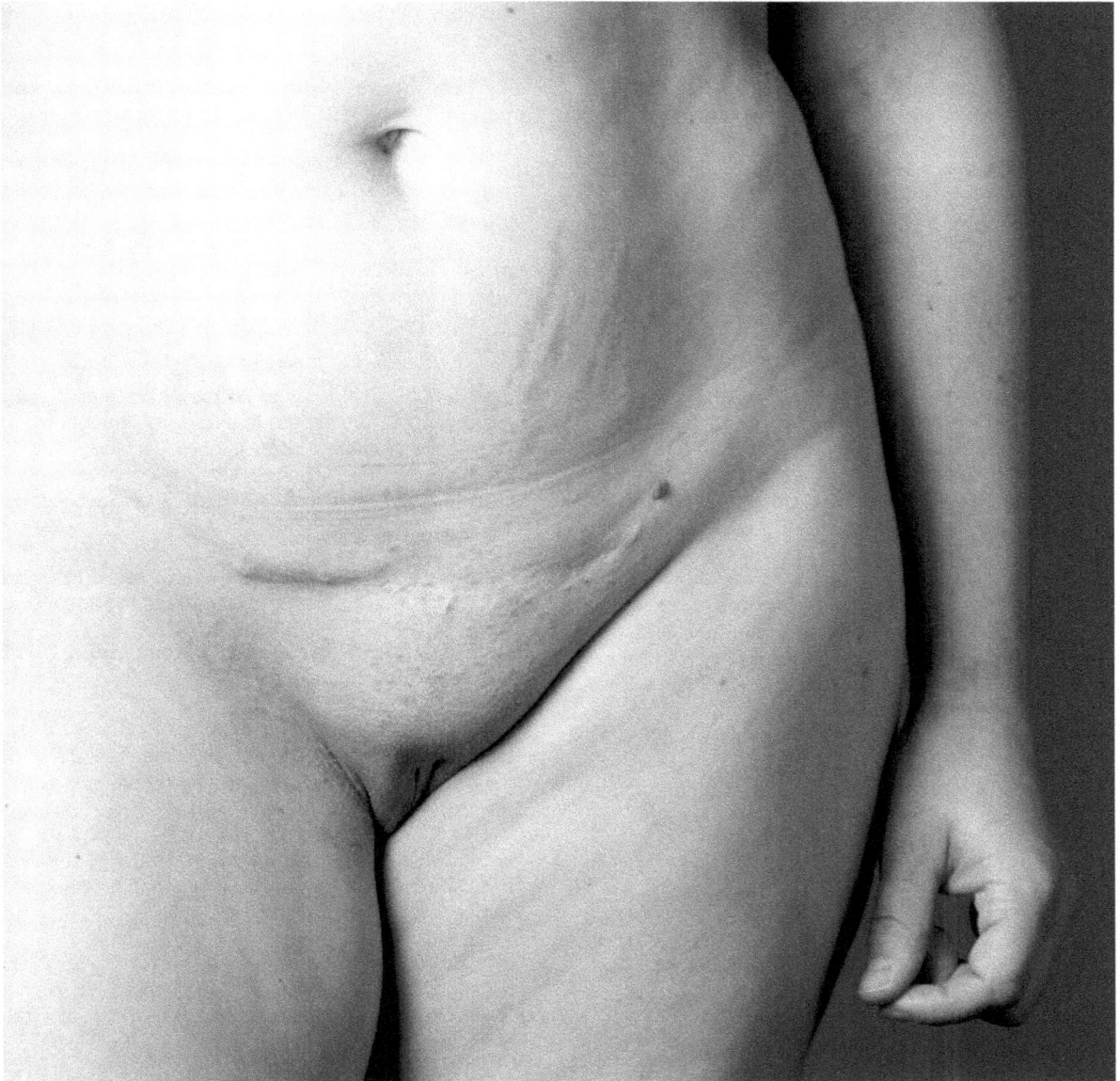

Caesarean mothers with three sections

[T001]   The Caesarean section is an operation, a trauma:

And women I know would have preferred normal births. My three sisters and I have 8 children between us. And all 8 children were delivered by section!! P.S. All of us were born "normally".

Occupation: Veterinary surgeon.

When I hear the word "Caesarean section" the following words come to mind spontaneously: Being at someone's mercy, having failed, saving mother and child, not being able to have any more children, pain, unconsciousness.

The birth of my first child (first section): Contractions: No. Head circumference 38 cm, height 50 cm, weight 3680 g, duration of pregnancy: 40 weeks. Breech presentation, too risky with primipara, child had the umbilical cord wrapped around the neck twice.

The first intensive physical contact with my first child: Approx. 1 hour after the operation.

I had problems breastfeeding after the first Caesarean: Difficulties with the breast (bleeding nipple, galactostasis), child did not gain weight. I breastfed for more than 1 year.

The birth of my second child (second section): Natural contractions: Approx. 20 hours. Induced labour: Approx. 23 hours. Head circumference 35.5 cm, height 54 cm, weight 3830 g, duration of pregnancy: 41 weeks. It is not possible to describe this birth briefly. It was a "chemical birth".

The second section had the following indication: "Cephalopelvic disproportion" or rather "patient-obstetrician/midwife disproportion".

Prior to the second Caesarean I received drugs: Everything: Tocolytics, "Synto drip", epidural, general anaesthetic.

The second Caesarean proceeded without complications: I do not know the surgical report, was under general anaesthetic.

The very first eye-contact with my second child: Approx. 8 hours after the operation?

The first intensive physical contact with my second child: Approx. 10 hours after the operation?

The birth of my third child (third section): Contractions: No. Head circumference 36.5 cm, height 50 cm, weight 3430 g, duration of pregnancy: 40 weeks. After two Caesareans normally a third one is performed, risk is too high because of scars.

The indication for my third section: Second repeat Caesarean section.

I had health problems after my three Caesarean sections: Disc prolapses, operation of intervertebral disc, weight problems, depression.

I would have preferred natural (vaginal) births: Yes.

I experienced the three Caesarean births as traumatic: Not the first or the third but the second.

The Caesarean was the ideal way of giving birth as far as I am concerned: No.

A Caesarean possibly has negative effects on the child: Traumatised mothers traumatise their children: The effects only become apparent later on.

Due to the following the rate of Caesareans is rising: People think women are not capable of giving birth, women don't think they are capable of doing it themselves, cutting is done too quickly.

My fundamental attitude on the topic "Caesarean": Lifesaving surgery has degenerated into a cosmetic "trifle". Birth considered to be an "illness" becomes "healthy" surgery.

My Caesarean scar (length approx. 20 cm):

With the first child I could not accept the fact of being "cut open" horizontally. Part of the skin is "missing" and the abdomen has become an abhorrent part of my body. My Caesarean scar is ugly because the "old" scar was cut away with every further C-section and a new one was created on my abdomen by a man (gynaecologist)!

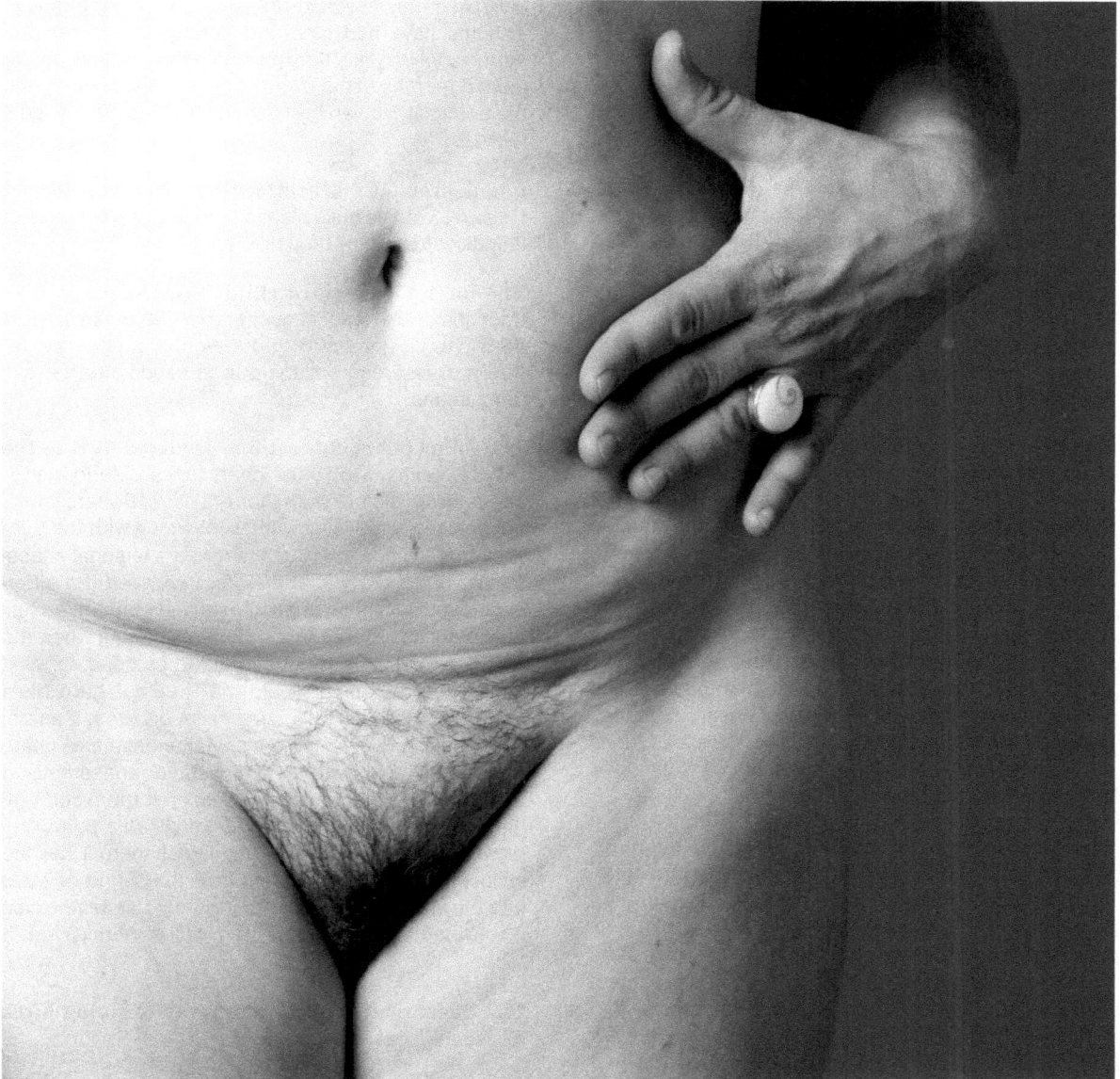

I had strong pain in the intestine (whole stomach, especially around the navel): Hellish back pain and radiating pain in the right leg [...]. Seven years later finally diagnosed as endometriosis (in my opinion due to the section). Since then many operations, consultations and constant pain for 17 years which is spreading continually.

Occupation: Employee.

When I hear the word "Caesarean section" the following words come to mind spontaneously: New life, pain, afterpains, emergency solution, botched life.

The birth of my first child (first section): Contractions: No. Head circumference 24 cm, height 34 cm, weight 880 g, duration of pregnancy: 30 weeks. Emergency Caesarean section due to severe preeclampsia (gestosis).

I had problems breastfeeding after the first Caesarean: I expressed milk and only needed very little because of the premature infant. I never breastfed.

The first Caesarean interfered with the mother-child bonding: The mother-child relationship had to be built up "artificially", there was no inner feeling! It was about our daughter surviving. As my condition was not too great the first few days (blood pressure) I only saw a photo of my daughter the next day and was only taken to the neonatal ward by wheelchair on the third day (only light touching and fondling possible). Intensive physical contact was only possible after two months (child in heated cot)! My daughter had and has serious problems (thank God not physical), she does not have an "inner clock", can't show feelings, does not want physical contact. ... but all of this is ascribed to the premature delivery.

The birth of my second child (second section): Natural contractions: Approx. 5 hours. Head circumference 34.5 cm, height 50 cm, weight 2880 g, duration of pregnancy: 38 weeks. Emergency Caesarean section, high blood pressure, not controlled by midwife! I think the second Caesarean could have been avoided: Midwife did not check on me and left me alone until it was too late and an emergency Caesarean section was performed. The "mother-child pass" of the first child was only checked after the operation, although I should have had strict monitoring (state after premature delivery/section/preeclampsia)! It took me at least 6 months to get over the severe disappointment, the animosity... Even my husband is still suffering (guilt feelings).

I had problems breastfeeding after the second Caesarean: The child slept a lot due to severe case of jaundice: tea – only breastfed for 14 days.

The birth of my third child (third section): Contractions: No. Head circumference 33.8 cm, height 48.5 cm, weight 2800 g, duration of pregnancy: 37 weeks. Caesarean section due to condition after two Caesareans.

The following complications occurred during the third Caesarean: Foetal heart tones deteriorated – anaesthesia did not work (horror!!) Now, 8 years later, I am only really realising what went wrong with the third section: [...] I do know that I received a regional anaesthesia, but not more. Therefore, I checked the difference between spinal anaesthesia and epidural anaesthesia online. There I found 5 points stating when the spinal anaesthesia is not allowed to be done: Existing damage of the spine! Could the "trauma" have been avoided? The hospital's surgery report says: General anaesthesia. Fact is, I had a spinal anaesthesia (state after L5-S1 laminectomy) and was not anaesthetised at all: I was able to move my legs, I felt the blood running out of the vagina, I felt unimaginable pain, I remember screaming, I was not quite all there, I saw the child, it was healthy, I crawled from the operating table into the sickbed by myself, therefore no anaesthesia... It was horrible for me and I am still suffering from it today.

The Caesarean was the ideal way of giving birth as far as I am concerned: No.

My Caesarean scars (length approx. 12 cm):

Very thin, very nice, hardly visible (despite three sections) – but can be felt! One only sees the scar on the outside. But the inner scars and the mental pain are felt. My Caesarean scars: "Beautiful on the outside – ugly on the inside!"

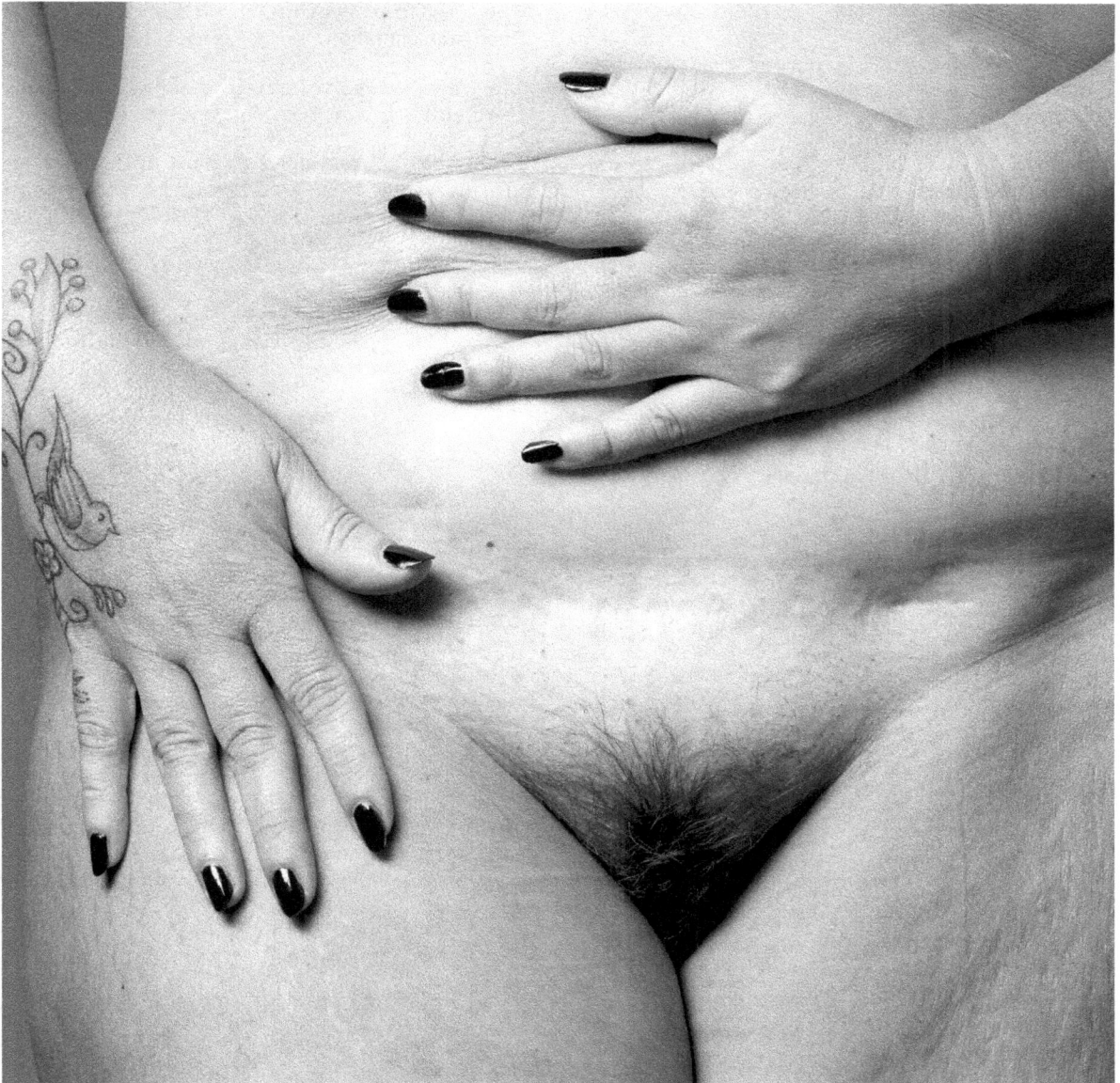

The Caesarean was the ideal way of giving birth as far as I am concerned:

After the second child I knew that another birth was not possible.

Occupation: Lawyer.

When I hear the word "Caesarean section" the following words come to mind spontaneously: n.s.

The birth of my first child (first section): Natural contractions: Approx. 9 hours. Head circumference 35 cm, height 51 cm, weight 3395 g, duration of pregnancy: 42 weeks. Preparation for natural birth, then after protracted duration of birth: Caesarean section. Pelvimetry and realisation that natural birth is impossible, pelvis too narrow.

The indication for my first section: Protracted labour.

The very first eye-contact and intensive physical contact with my first child: Approx. 12 hours after the operation.

The birth of my second child (second section): Natural contractions: Approx. 6 ½ hours. Head circumference 34 cm, height 52 cm, weight 2887 g, duration of pregnancy: 39 weeks. Repeat Caesarean section due to pelvis being too narrow.

My second child was injured through the Caesarean section: A very small cut on the cheek.

The very first eye-contact with my second child: During the operation.

The first intensive physical contact with my second child: Approx. 1 ½ hours after the operation.

The birth of my third child (third section): Natural contractions: Approx 4 ½ hours. Head circumference 33 cm, height 47 cm, weight 2740 g, duration of pregnancy: 38 weeks. Repeat Caesarean section due to pelvis being too narrow.

The very first eye-contact with my third child: During the operation.

The first intensive physical contact with my third child: Approx. 1 ½ hours after the operation.

I was able to breastfeed without difficulty after all three Caesareans: I breastfed for more than six months each time.

The Caesareans interfered with the mother-child bonding: No.

I would have preferred natural (vaginal) births: With the first birth yes.

I was afraid of pain during birth/of perineal trauma: No.

I miss having a natural birth experience: No.

Society gives me the feeling of having failed: No.

I find that Caesarean section is trivialised and minimised by the media (newspaper, magazines, television, ...): Partly yes, since a Caesarean section with its consequences is comparable to any other surgery (and it definitely takes time to recover from it).

Due to the following the rate of Caesareans is rising: Fixed date, fear of pain and natural birth.

My fundamental attitude on the topic "Caesarean": In my case the only way to deliver children. Generally an alternative to "natural birth" for all those, who need one, whatever the case may be.

My Caesarean scar (length approx. 18 cm):

My Caesarean scar healed without a problem. I treated my Caesarean scar with scar ointment. It looks like a smiling mouth.

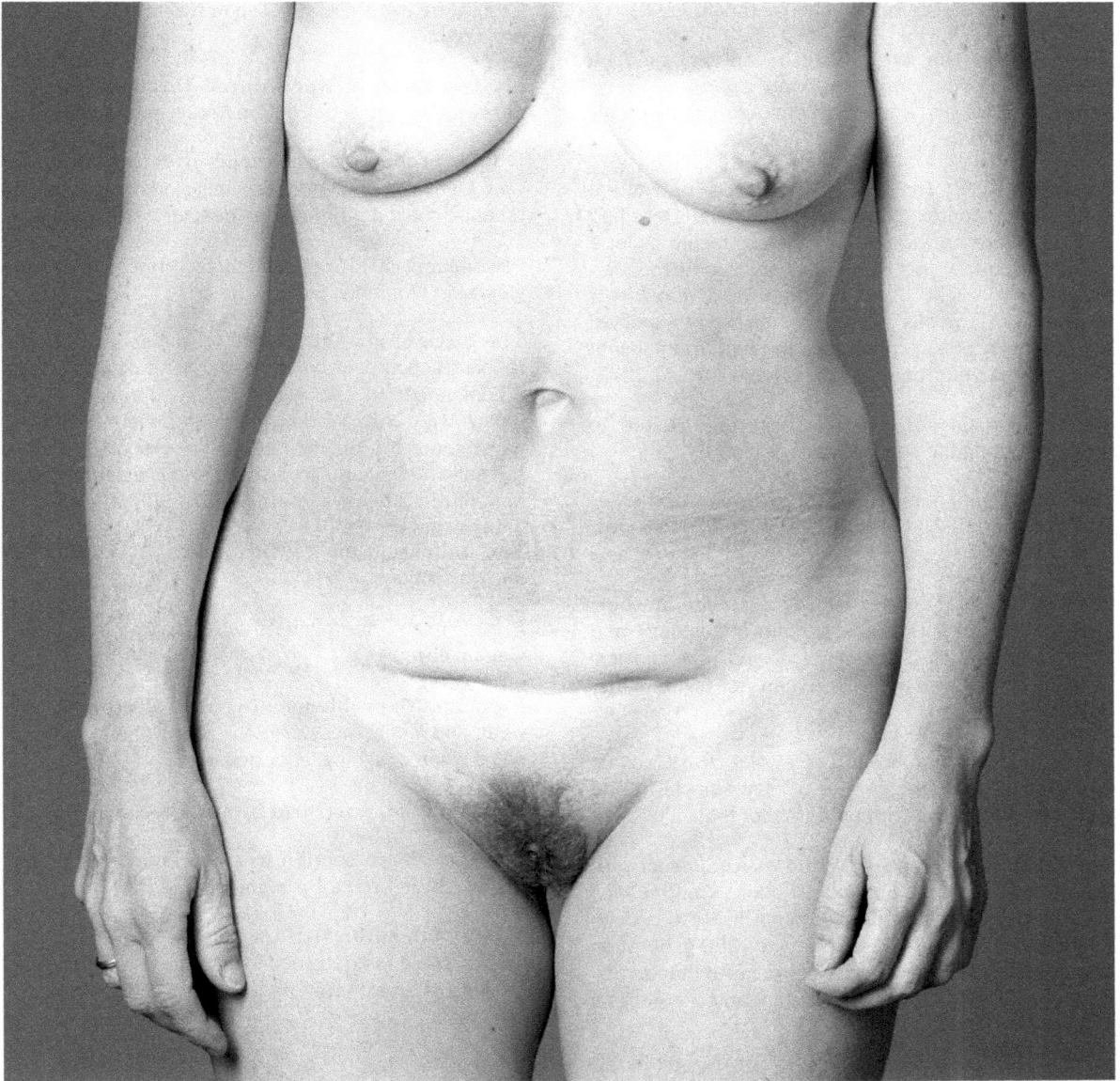

a cut which brought
my children into life;
a cut into my
womanliness,

scars on my body,
scars on my soul.
A cut in my life – I will never
be the same again.

But still
a cut which brought
my children
into life.

Occupation: Registered Speech Therapist.

When I hear the word "Caesarean section" the following words come to mind spontaneously: Pain, trauma, scars, abdominal operation, cut – on my body, in my life.

The birth of my first child (first section): Natural contractions: Approx. 17 hours. Contractions intensified by drugs: Duration unknown. I received tocolytics for a while then labour was induced again. Head circumference 34 cm, height 52 cm, weight 3560 g, duration of pregnancy: 40 weeks +6 days. I had never expected the possibility of a section, was (and am) traumatised! Epidural was unfortunately not possible.

The indication for my first section: Failure to progress during the second stage of labour.

I had problems breastfeeding after the first Caesarean: Not enough milk, no support. Pain due to section!

The first Caesarean interfered with the mother-child bonding: Due to the general anaesthetic and pain I was in such a bad physical and psychological condition that I was not able to care for my daughter the way I wanted to.

I suffered from depression after the first Caesarean: Started suddenly on the 3rd day after birth and lasted for weeks. Was not prepared for that.

The birth of my second child (second section): Natural contractions: Approx. 10 hours. Contractions intensified by drugs: Duration unknown. Head circumference 34 cm, height 55 cm, weight 4050 g, duration of pregnancy: 40 weeks. Was very relieved that an epidural was possible, on no account wanted a general anaesthesia again.

The indication for my second section: Failure to progress.

My second child was injured through the Caesarean section: Small cut on the back by scalpel.

I had problems breastfeeding after the second Caesarean: Hardly any milk, hard, very painful breasts, could not breastfeed despite best support.

My second child has health problems now: Allergies, skin problems.

The birth of my third child (third section): Natural contractions: Approx 5 hours. Head circumference 33 cm, height 51 cm, weight 3210 g, duration of pregnancy: 37 weeks +4 days. Sudden onset of labour 6 days before the planned section – everything had to go really fast again. Nevertheless, this was the "most beautiful" birth.

The indication for my third section: Condition after two sections.

I had problems breastfeeding after the third Caesarean: Yes.

I had health problems after my Caesareans: Very weak abdominal muscles: Back pain when lying down, pains when coughing, sneezing, etc.

I miss having a natural birth experience: Yes.

The Caesarean section was the ideal way of giving birth as far as I am concerned: No.

My fundamental attitude on the topic "Caesarean": I would restrict a section to a medical indication, the idea of an elective Caesarean section is strange.

My Caesarean scars (length approx. 13 cm):

I had my Caesarean scars treated with osteopathy. I feel my Caesarean
scars as follows: Paraesthesia between scars and navel.

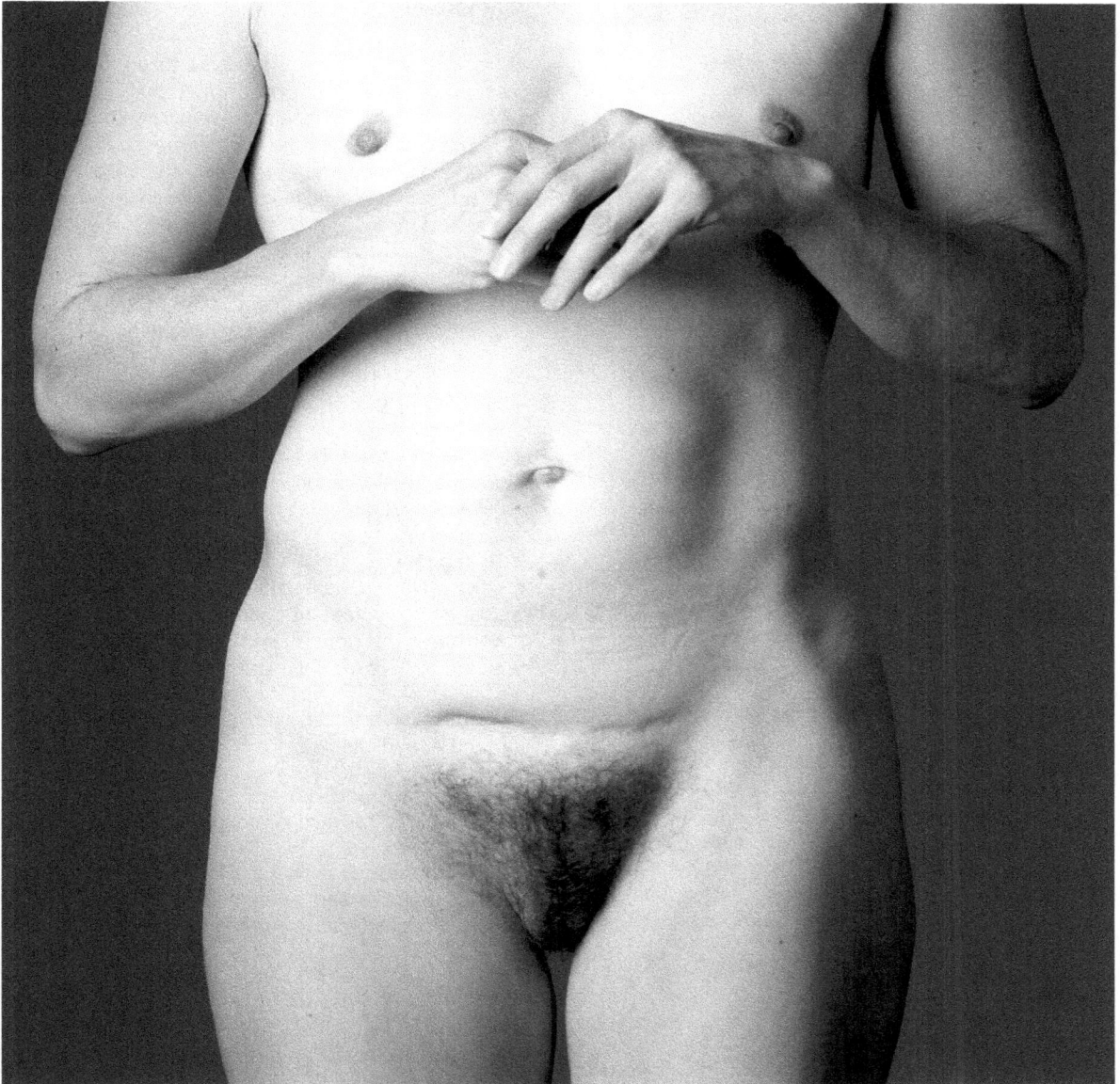

[T088]   My second child:

died 20 hours after birth.

Occupation: Innkeeper.

When I hear the word "Caesarean section" the following words come to mind spontaneously: Insecurity, fear, failure, not being part of the crowd, scar.

The birth of my first child (first section): Natural contractions: Approx. 5 hours. Contractions induced by drugs: Approx. 9 hours. Head circumference 36 cm, height 54 cm, weight 3820 g, duration of pregnancy: 41 weeks. I got pregnant at the age of 32. We waited for this child for four years. Two months before I had finally given up ever getting pregnant. After 10 hours of intensive contractions I could not accept a Caesarean section. Total disappointment.

The indication for my first section: High stage I.p.

The first Caesarean interfered with the mother-child bonding: Due to the anaesthesia I thought I was still pregnant. I had severe pain in my abdomen and thought I was still in labour.

My second child: Surprisingly pregnant again, prepared for a normal birth till the end.

I was afraid of pain during birth/of perineal trauma: No, but of injury to the scar.

The birth of my second child (second section): Natural contractions: Approx. 3 hours. Head circumference 37 cm, height 53 cm, weight 4120 g, duration of pregnancy: 41 weeks +3 days. I was already 10 days overdue, when a Caesarean was planned because of the high position of the child. Hours before, contractions began. In the room next door three children were born normally that night. I cried and wished so badly it would drop, I thought I felt that it wanted to come out at the bottom now. I received tocolytics and the planned Caesarean [...] [with an epidural] so I could witness the birth. I hoped he would make it through the night because I felt the engorgement of my breasts and my body preparing for feeding the child. Through a mouthful of amniotic fluid mixed with meconium, the veins clotted and the blood circulated in the reverse direction. [corrected by Dr. Förster: Through inhaling meconium raised lung pressure with changed circulation of the blood.] My son died after 20 hours and for the first time in my life I felt endless pain.

My third child: I lost this child in the 7th week without even knowing that I had ever had it.

My fourth child: This pregnancy was a seesaw of emotions and fears, physically ideal, did not gain too much weight. Planned Caesarean section.

The birth of my fourth child (third section): Contractions: No. Head circumference n.s., height 51 cm, weight 3466 g, duration of pregnancy: 38 weeks. I will never forget the first touch of my child on the cheek! With the birth of my daughter I started living again.

The indication for my third section: High-risk birth for mother and child.

A Caesarean birth possibly has negative effects on the child: The child is yanked out of the belly.

My fundamental attitude on the topic "Caesarean": If a Caesarean section is necessary then it is best for the child and the mother.

My Caesarean scar (length approx. 11 cm):

I think that I feel less energy in my lower abdomen due to the Caesarean and
that I, therefore, also have less desire for sex. I only realised this years later.

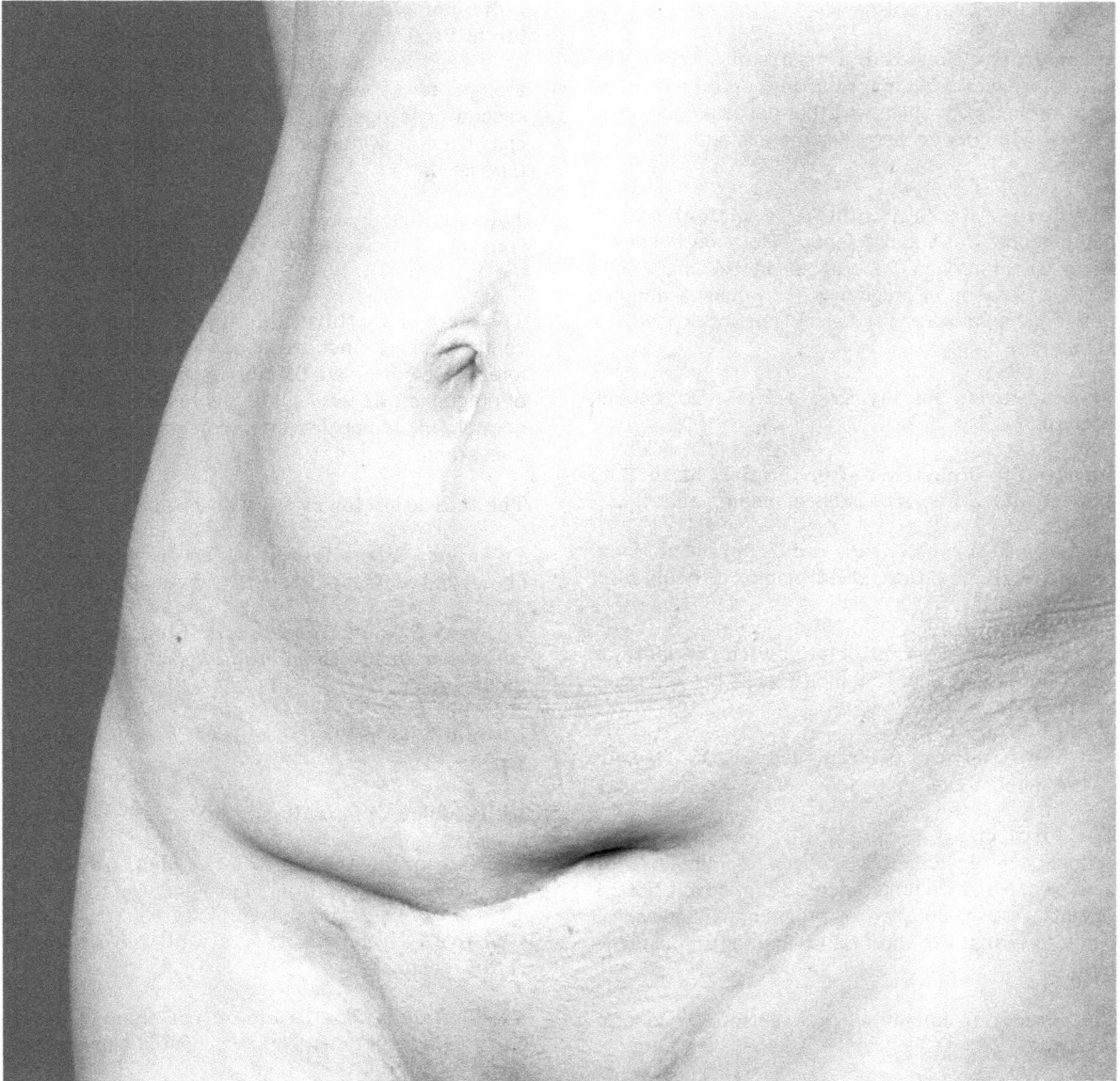

Caesarean mothers with three sections

[T003] Back then the transverse cut just became fashionable:

I was appalled by my long scar.

Occupation: Telephonist.

When I hear the word "Caesarean section" the following words come to mind spontaneously: Poor mother, poor child, was that necessary?, a topic that will hopefully be discussed more in antenatal education.

The birth of my first child (first section): Natural contractions: No. Induced labour: Duration unknown. Head circumference 36 cm, height 54 cm, weight 4310 g, duration of pregnancy: 43 weeks. 2 minutes before 8 the Caesarean is decided on. Shock. I feel the cut and the pain.

The indication for my first section: Not enough contractions.

I wanted to breastfeed after the first birth: But I stopped after 4 weeks because of inflammations.

The very first eye-contact and intensive physical contact with my first child: Approx. 5 hours after the operation.

The first Caesarean interfered with the mother-child bonding: Because it took a while before I could see my child.

My first child was injured through the Caesarean: A minimal scar in the face.

The birth of my second child (second section): Natural contractions: No. Induced labour: Duration unknown. Head circumference 35 cm, height 50 cm, weight 3600 g, duration of pregnancy: 41 weeks. I came to terms with the first Caesarean through this birth.

The indication for my second section: No contractions.

I did not want to breastfeed after the second birth: Because of the bad experiences with my first child I did not breastfeed my second child. I would though, advise every mother to try it again with the second child despite bad experiences with the first child because with me it worked out perfectly with my third child.

The very first eye-contact and intensive physical contact with my second child: Approx. 2 hours after the operation.

The birth of my third child (third section): Natural contractions: No. Induced labour: Maybe. Head circumference 36 cm, height 52 cm, weight 3800 g, duration of pregnancy: 41 weeks. I hoped to be able to deliver normally but the obstetrician immediately scheduled a Caesarean.

The indication for my third section: n.s.

I wanted to breastfeed after the third Caesarean: I breastfed without a problem for a couple of months.

The very first eye-contact and intensive physical contact with my third child: Approx. 2 hours after the operation.

I would have preferred natural (vaginal) births: Yes.

I was afraid of pain during birth: Yes.

The Caesarean section was the ideal way of giving birth as far as I am concerned: No.

Due to the following the rate of Caesareans is rising: I cannot say.

My fundamental attitude on the topic "Caesarean": In case of emergency: yes. Out of convenience: no.

My Caesarean scar (length approx. 15 cm):

My abdomen is split into two parts, definitely not nice. I felt my Caesarean scar for about 15 years with weather changes or pressure from zips. In the meantime I have managed to accept my Caesarean scar.

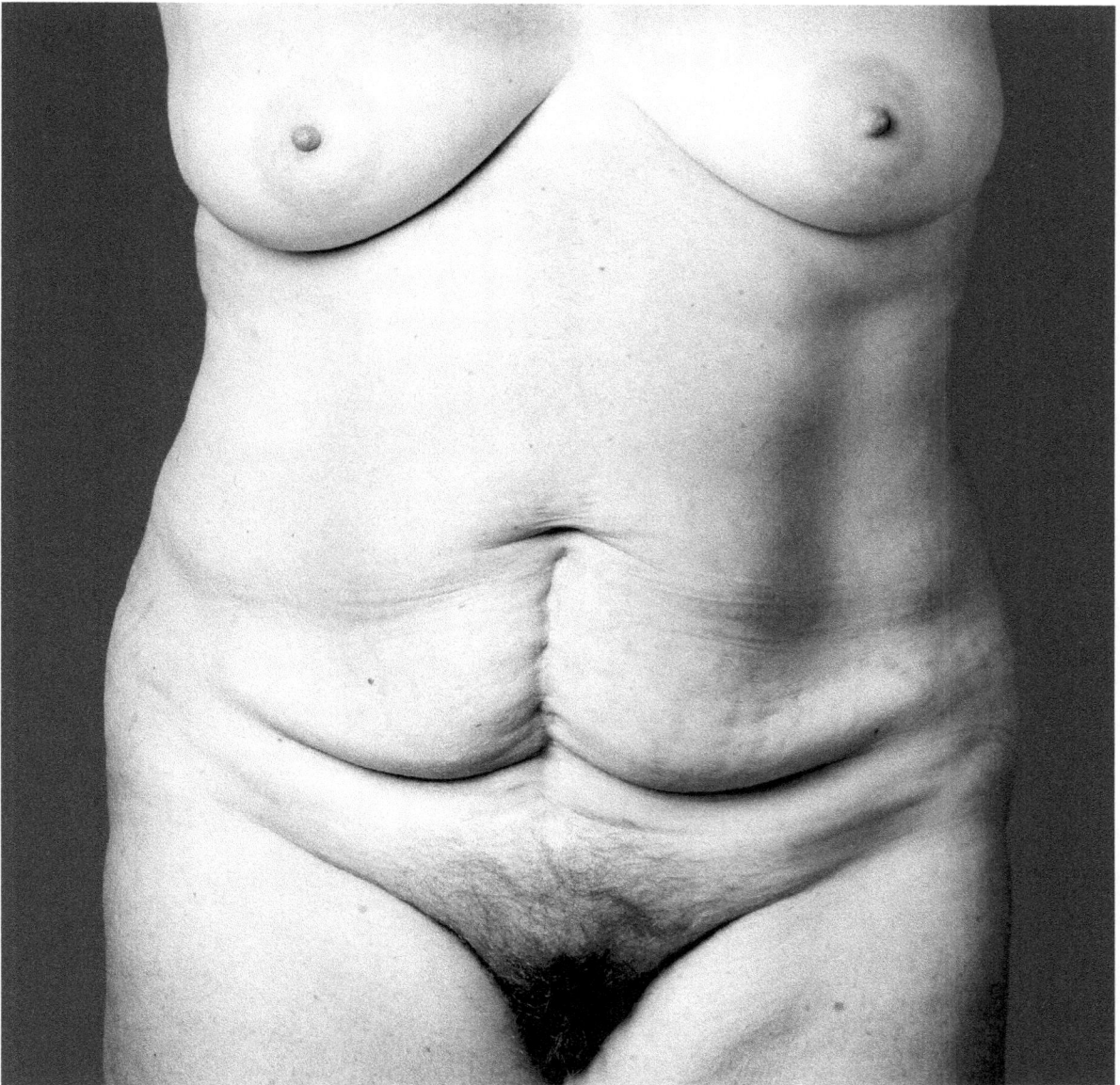

Caesarean mothers with three sections

Caesarean mothers with four sections

Accompanied by great fear, everything went well though!

Occupation: At the moment housewife.

When I hear the word "Caesarean section" the following words come to mind spontaneously: Fear, pain, disappointment, being at someone's mercy or being helpless, psychodrama (my husband says!!).

The birth of my first child (first section): Natural contractions: Approx. 20 hours. Induced labour: Approx. 15 hours. Head circumference 35 cm, height 53 cm, weight 3650 g, duration of pregnancy: 41 weeks. After 39 hours in the delivery room – emergency Caesarean section. A nightmare!

The indication for my first section: Drop in foetal heart rate.

The first intensive physical contact with my first child: Approx. 8 to 9 hours after the operation.

The first Caesarean interfered with the mother-child bonding: When I saw her for the first time, approx. 3 ½ hours after the operation, my daughter was screaming. I was not capable of taking her – just not capable!

I had problems breastfeeding after the first Caesarean: Raw nipples, inflammation of the breast.

The birth of my second child (second section): Natural contractions: Duration unknown. Head circumference 37 cm, height 55 cm, weight 3885 g, duration of pregnancy: 41 weeks. Long but "normal" birth up to the pushing contractions, but then cephalopelvic disproportion.

The indication for my second section: Cephalopelvic disproportion.

My partner was present during the second Caesarean and stood by me: No, he died in an accident 7 weeks before the birth.

The birth of my third child (third section): Contractions: No. Head circumference 32.5 cm, height 52 cm, weight 2860 g, duration of pregnancy: 37 weeks. Planned Caesarean section – first birth that proceeded positively (no complications).

The indication for my third section: Had had 2 Caesareans already – no other possibility?

The birth of my fourth child (fourth section): Contractions: No. Head circumference 35 cm, height 50 cm, weight 3020 g, duration of pregnancy: 38 weeks.

The indication for my fourth section: 3 previous Caesareans.

I would have preferred natural (vaginal) births: Yes.

The Caesarean section was the ideal way of giving birth as far as I am concerned: No.

Due to the following the rate of Caesareans is rising: Due to trivialising propaganda a lot of people are unaware that it is "major surgery".

My fundamental attitude on the topic "Caesarean": I am thankful that this medical alternative allows one to have healthy children if there is no other possibility. But never as an alternative to normal birth!

My Caesarean scar (length approx. 20 cm):

With the first and second birth the abdominal area was cut open, with the third and fourth birth only a part was cut and the rest ripped. I have a very numb feeling around the navel. Burning pain when touched. After physio-therapy it got a little better but the feeling stayed. My physician said that this was normal because the nerves had been cut through so many times.

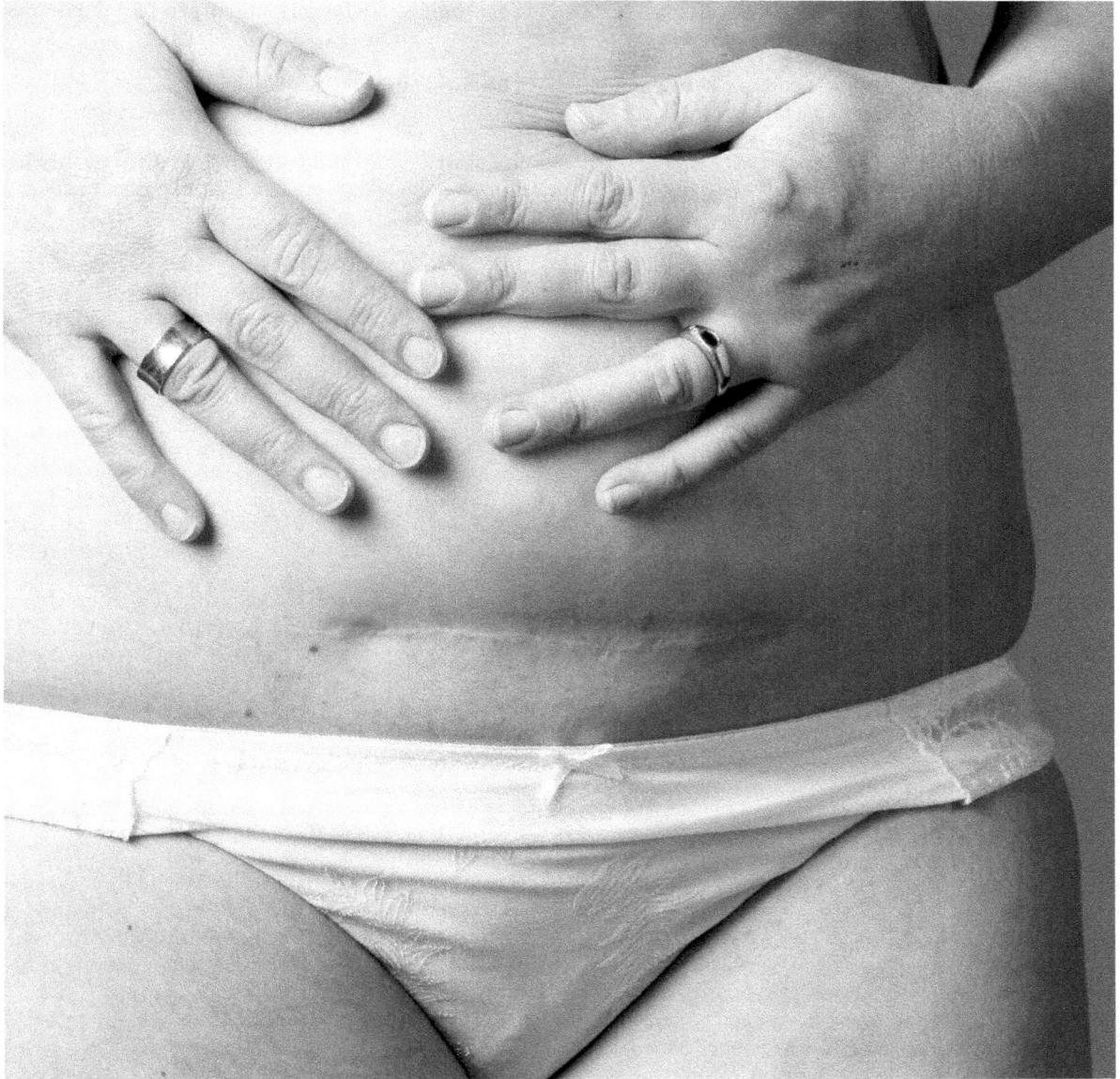

Partly.

Occupation: Clerical assistant

When I hear the word "Caesarean section" the following words come to mind spontaneously: Surgery, Caesarean scar, rising number of C-sections, "fashionable" – future of birth?

I dealt with Caesareans intensively prior to my first Caesarean birth: No. Was unfortunately also a "taboo topic" in antenatal class.

The birth of my first child (first section): Natural contractions: Approx. 48 hours. Induced labour: Approx. 3 hours. Head circumference 34 cm, height 53 cm, weight 3980 g, duration of pregnancy: 40 weeks. Short phase of "mourning" because of the "missed" birth experience of a spontaneous delivery.

The indication for my first section: Pathological CTG, secondary uterine insufficiency.

I suffered from depression after the first Caesarean: Feeling of having failed for a few hours – approx. one day after the surgery.

The birth of my second child (second section): Natural contractions: Approx. 7 hours. Head circumference 35 cm, height 52 cm, weight 3580 g, duration of pregnancy: 38 weeks. Something already familiar which repeats itself at intervals of one year, I have come to terms with it.

The indication for my second section: The timeframe between the first and the second section was too short (1 year).

The birth of my third child (third section): Natural contractions: Approx. 12 hours. Head circumference 37 cm, height 53 cm, weight 3740 g, duration of pregnancy: 38 weeks. Already routine, but shocked about hospital stay (2 days) due to adaptive difficulties of my child.

The indication for my third section: 2 previous sections – always a section.

The first intensive physical contact with my third child: Approx. 48 hours after the operation.

My third child had serious health problems: Adaptive difficulties (breathing) after birth – paediatric clinic.

The birth of my fourth child (fourth section): Contractions: No. Head circumference 35 cm, height 52 cm, weight 3180 g, duration of pregnancy: 36 weeks. Everything well-known, even hospitalisation due to premature adaptive difficulties not really mentally a problem.

The indication for my fourth section: 3rd repeat Caesarean section.

My fourth child had serious health problems: Adaptive difficulties with breathing, premature birth.

I was able to breastfeed without difficulty after all four Caesareans: I breastfed for a couple of months or for more than one year. I am still breastfeeding.

Due to the following the rate of Caesareans is rising: Scheduling, fear of pain during birth.

The Caesarean section was the ideal way of giving birth as far as I am concerned: No.

My fundamental attitude on the topic "Caesarean": Section should actually only be performed if there is a medical indication, elective Caesarean section only after sufficient, sound information and not frivolously.

My Caesarean scar (length approx. 14 cm):

My Caesarean scar is red at the moment, a little bulging.
Maybe I should try some scar ointment.

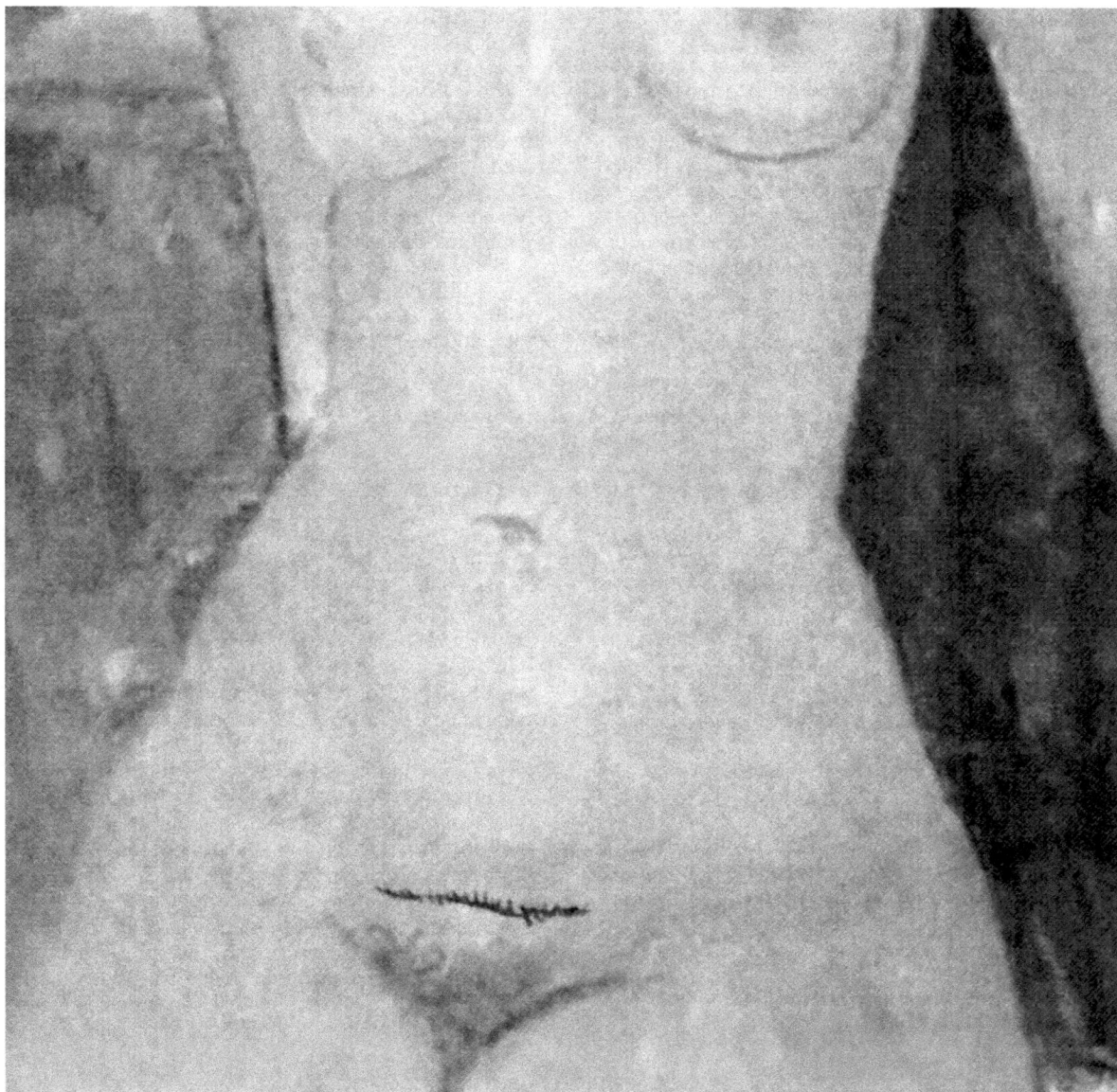

With my 5 children having been delivered by Caesarean section. I do not feel inferior or incapable but like a "fully-fledged" woman and mother.

Occupation: Medical assistant/secretary

When I hear the word "Caesarean section" the following words come to mind spontaneously: Relief, joy, excitement, finally!, fear.

The birth of my first child (first section): Natural contractions: Approx. 30 hours. Head circumference 35 cm, height 53 cm, weight 4400 g, duration of pregnancy: 41 weeks. Difficult delivery, after many hours of contractions and no result (cervical dilatation only a few centimetres) – Caesarean section.

The indication for my first section: Unfavourable cervix, mother and child exhausted.

The birth of my second child (second section): Contractions: No. Head circumference 37 cm, height 54 cm, weight 4850 g, duration of pregnancy: 37 weeks. Waters broke 2 weeks before term.

The indication for my second section: Premature rupture of membranes and previous section without contractions.

The birth of my third child (third section): Contractions: No. Head circumference 37 cm, height 52 cm, weight 4470 g, duration of pregnancy: 38 weeks. Planned Caesarean section – 2 weeks before term.

The indication for my third section: My age, two existing Caesarean sections.

The birth of my fourth and fifth child (twins, fourth section): Natural contractions: A couple of days. Head circumference 33.5/36 cm, height 51/51 cm, weight 3010/3510 g, duration of pregnancy: 35 weeks +2 days.

The indication for my fourth section: My age, twins, three existing sections.

Prior to the fourth Caesarean I received drugs: Medication to slow down labour.

I did not breastfeed after any of the four Caesareans: I was not patient enough after the first one, after the other three Caesareans I did not want to breastfeed at all.

My children had health problems / have health problems now: No.

I would have preferred natural (vaginal) births: With the first and the second birth yes, but with the third and the fourth birth not anymore.

I was afraid of pain during birth/of perineal trauma: Yes.

The Caesarean section was the ideal way of giving birth as far as I am concerned: No.

Due to the following the rate of Caesareans is rising: Many women may think that it is less painful or easier to deliver children by Caesarean section.

My fundamental attitude on the topic "Caesarean": I find that there is too much negative talk about the Caesarean birth. We are told normal birth is the best (might be true). But it should also be seen as a gift to be able to have healthy children despite problems like a narrow pelvis, large children, no strength. Nowadays, one almost has to be ashamed of having Caesarean children. "Something must be wrong with that woman not being able to manage a normal birth". I am proud of my children, of the births and the pregnancies. I think it is most important to feel fine and start caring for the child during pregnancy (no smoking, drinking etc.), one must start then to love and take time to stroke one's tummy. Giving love, warmth and comfort after the birth of the children is indispensable to life for both mother and child. It is secondary then whether the child entered the world "normally" or by Caesarean section.

My Caesarean scar (length approx. 19 cm):

I can feel my Caesarean scar as follows: Numbness.
It is flat and has the shape of a half moon.

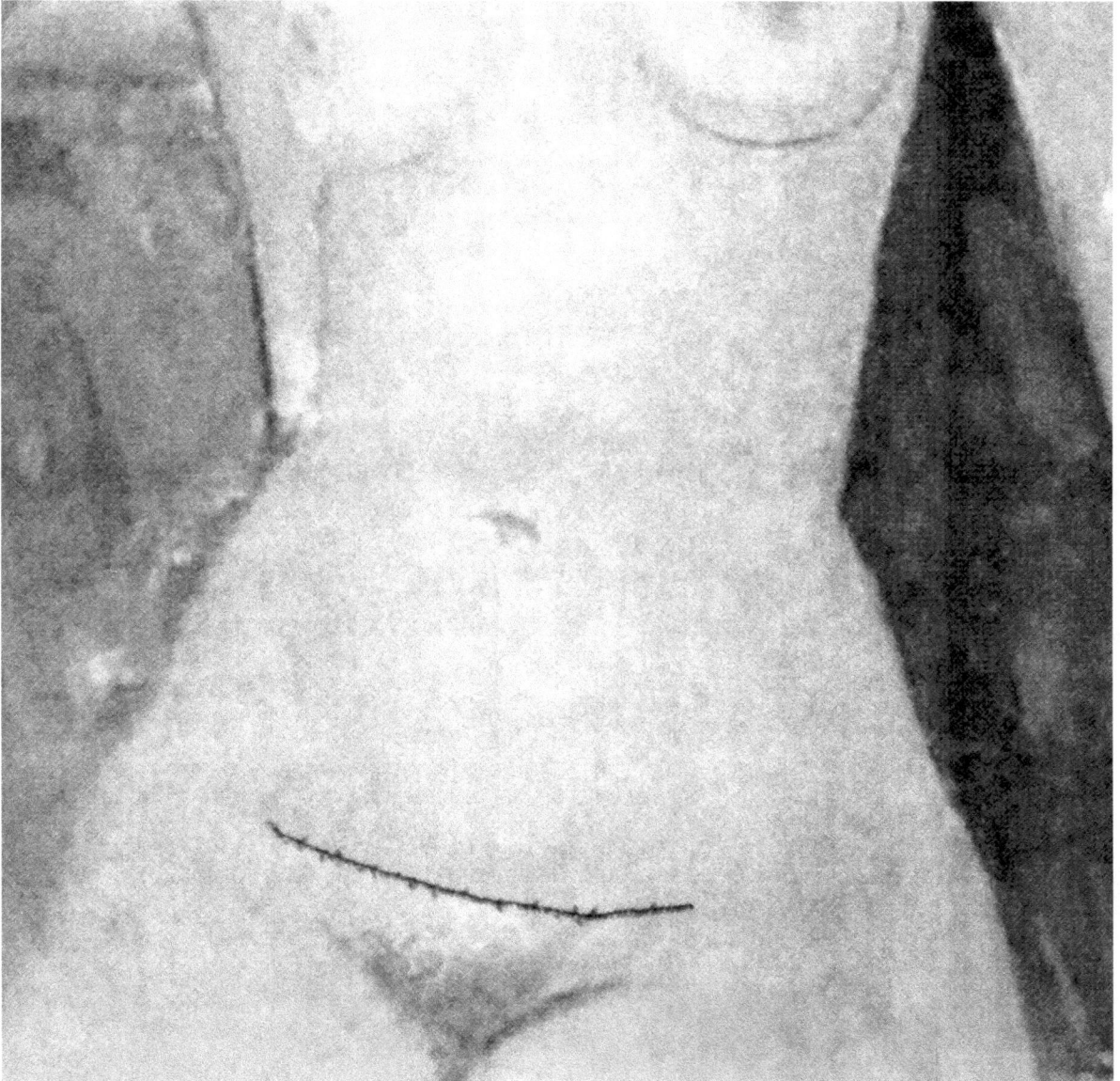

Caesarean mothers with four sections

The "gentle Caesarean section"

Photo report of a Caesarean section using the "Misgav Ladach" method

A "Caesarean section" (simplified theoretical description)

Both straight abdominal muscles (rectus abdominis muscles) are mostly just pulled apart, not cut; they can tear unintentionally though.

Schematically drawn "Caesarean section" (white line)

The penetrated layers of the body from the outside to the inside:

1 Skin (Dermis)
2 Subcutaneous tissue (Subcutis)
3 Superficial fascia
4 Abdominal muscles / aponeurosis / fascia
5 Internal abdominal fascia
6 Median peritoneum fold
7 Peritoneum
8 Uterus

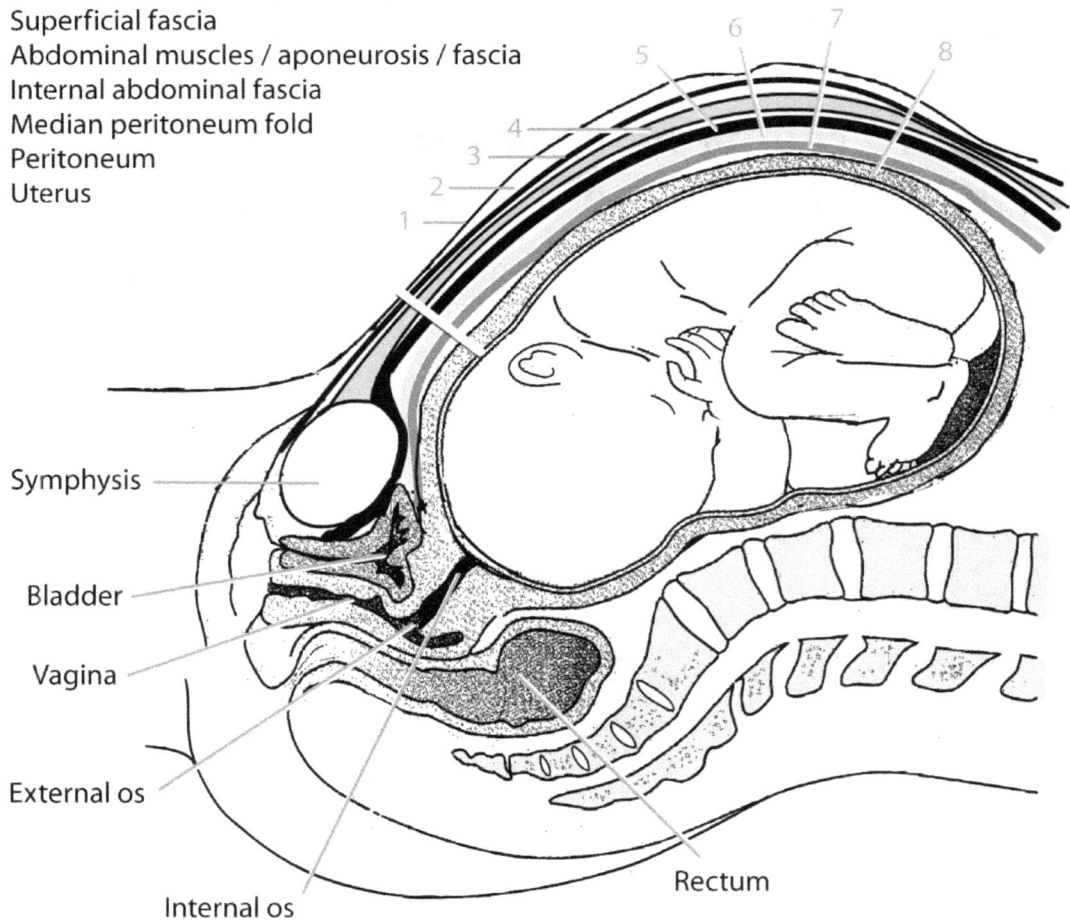

The "gentle Caesarean section" – is there really such a thing? Our photographer Gudrun Wesp went in search of it in spring 2006 and captured, in numerous photographs, a Misgav Ladach section, which was performed at a clinic in the province of Salzburg. We forwent displaying the photos in colour – because of the black-and-white concept of the book, as well as to go easy on the faint-hearted.

We want to, hereby, thank participant T010 who not only let us take photos of her before and after the surgery but also allowed us to attend the scheduled Caesarean section of her third child in agreement with the clinic (Indication: Condition after two previous Caesareans).

Before we explain every one of the photos shown and subsequently display the photo report, we want to look at how "gentle" major abdominal surgery, as in the case of a Caesarean section, can actually be and what the frequently heard name "Misgav Ladach" means. Volker Lehmann tells us the following on this subject in his book "The Imperial Cut. The History of an Operation" (Schattauer, Stuttgart 2006), which is definitely worth reading:

"Concealed behind the phrase "gentle Caesarean section" is a procedure which can only seldom be evaluated by patients but is supposed to give them a comforting sensation, a sense of well-being towards the operation. The procedure itself is not as new as it seems to be. The skin is cut through with a scalpel in exactly the same way as in the case of a classic Caesarean section. Even in the past the adipose tissue was pulled aside from the fascia with blunt hooks and in the same way the bellies of the rectus abdominis muscle were pulled apart. The blunt extension of the small sharp incision in the uterine wall was already described by Kehrer when he did his first Caesarean section [...] in 1881. Therefore, what the gentle section promises is not very new nor very gentle. It is doubtful whether ripping is gentler than cutting and whether it should be described as such. The proclamation of the gentle Caesarean though

caused a new appraisal of the intensive post-operative treatment of patients with drainages, bladder catheters, fasting and infusions, even although all these measures were not necessary with the conventional section but were performed by surgeons anyway. The gentle Caesarean section is actually called the Misgav Ladach method. This term does not make it easy for clinics to win patients as customers, therefore it was called the "gentle Caesarean section". Misgav Ladach is a hospital in Jerusalem. There this method, which is not totally new in its individual stages, was compiled and published by M. Stark in 1994. It should be an operating technique which requires few instruments, simple movements and very little after-treatment. In Jerusalem the idea was not to make up for dwindling numbers in patients but being able to manage with few instruments and little sewing material." (Translated English version from the original German book, page 231)

Despite this matter-of-fact account of obviously invasive surgery the "Misgav-Ladach method of a section" is repeatedly propagated as the "gentle Caesarean section".

Every reader should decide on his/her own whether, and if so, how gentle a "Caesarean section" is for mother and child. [Number of picture] and time are based upon the digital camera used for these photographs.

01 [7051] 7:32 a.m.

Just after half past seven in the morning the operating theatre is still deserted. The patient will later receive oxygen and the anaesthetic gas from the anaesthetic equipment.

02 [7069] 7:48 a.m.

The instruments for the upcoming Caesarean section are placed ready: About 40 scissors, tweezers, clamps, retractors and needles will be used.

03 [7082] 7:56 a.m.

The surgeon's hands which are covered with long plastic gloves examine the pregnant woman's abdomen once again. Her abdomen is covered with a sterile plastic sheet which has a reddish shimmer. A construction which looks like a hoop holds a circular plastic cover in position. If, later on, amniotic fluid or blood should leak out of the abdomen nothing will run out uncontrolled over the operating table. Furthermore, the patient remains clean and dry.

04 [7093] 8:02 a.m.

The surgeon marks the position of the section, the so-called "Pfannenstiel incision" while his assistant holds the cover in place. The exact incision is of major importance for the smooth progression of the operation. In this case it is important to cut exactly into the previous scar of the first two Caesareans, but under no circumstances to cut into a varicose vein adjoining the old scar.

05 [7099] 8:03 a.m.

The incision is done accurately with a scalpel – it is a planned and not a quick emergency section. → Clearly visible: the marked varicose vein on the right hand side of the picture.

06 [7105] 8:04 a.m.

The transverse incision ("bikini cut") is approx. 15 cm long. → The subcutaneous tissue is visible.

07 [7113] 8:04 a.m.

The muscle fascia is dissected. → The connection of the rectus abdominis muscles becomes visible in the abdominal wall.

08 [7114] 8:05 a.m.

To be able to section the muscles lengthwise the surgeon has to separate the fascia on the left and the right from the muscle. In the case of a section performed according to the Misgav-Ladach method this is done with the fingers. In the past it used to be done with tweezers and scissors.

09 [7117] 8:05 a.m.

By displacing skin and fascia the surgeon creates a cavity.

10 [7130] 8:06 a.m.

The basic structure of the linea alba becomes visible.

11 [7138] 8:06 a.m.

The abdominal muscles are now separated and pulled apart, the peritoneum is open and the anterior wall of the uterus is visible. The abdominal wall is pulled apart with two retractors.

12 [7140] 8:07 a.m.

The uterus is now visible deep down.

13 [7154] 8:08 a.m.

An incision, approx. 5 cm in length, has been made in the uterus. While the assistant is still pulling the abdominal wall apart with the two retractors, the surgeon has placed both his index fingers inside the wound and is extending the incision with these.

14 [7156] 8:08 a.m.

Opening of the uterus four fingers in length and two fingers in width, which means a maximum of 12 to 13 cm, results in an opening with a diameter of 8.5 cm at most.

15 [7170] 8:08 a.m.

While the assistant holds the incision open on the left the surgeon pulls the abdominal wall upwards and places his left hand inside the womb to direct the child's head outwards. The assistant places his left hand on the fundus uteri to apply (contraction-like) pressure from that spot if instructed to do so by the surgeon.

16 [7175] 8:08 a.m.

The surgeon's left hand is inside the uterus mobilising the child's presenting part of the body (in this case the head) so that this can slide outwards on his hand.

17 [7186] 8:08 a.m.

Assistant and surgeon swap position of their hands: The surgeon is now applying pressure to the fundus uteri with his right hand while the assistant holds the upper edge of the wound slightly away with two fingers. Note: The assistant also often puts pressure on the fundus uteri and regulates it at the instruction of the surgeon.

18 [7187] 8:08 a.m.

Regulated, ...

19 [7188] 8:08 a.m.

slow expulsion ...

20 [7189] 8:09 a.m.

of the foetal head.

21 [7190] 8:09 a.m.

Now the surgeon grips the foetal head (performed in an identical manner by a midwife at a vaginal delivery) by placing the index finger on the occiput and the middle finger on the mandibula.

22 [7191] 8:09 a.m.

The head is lifted slightly with a regulated pull at the same time.

23 [7192] 8:09 a.m.

The right shoulder is visible (but not really born yet).

24 [7193] 8:09 a.m.

Now the foetal head is lowered with a regulated steady downward pull until the front (upper) shoulder, namely the left one, appears and ...

25 [7194] 8:09 a.m.

... the left shoulder is born completely. Note: This is the usual mechanism, imitated from nature: First the front (upper) shoulder is born by lowering the head, then by lifting the head is the back (lower) shoulder. Only in exceptional cases, when e.g. mobilising is difficult, the child is very large, the access too narrow etc., the back (lower) shoulder is born before the front (upper).

26 [7195] 8:09 a.m.

The surgeon's right hand grasps underneath the left foetal axilla, the surgeon's left hand underneath the right axilla. Steady regulated pulling.

27 [7197] 8:09 a.m.

Both foetal shoulders as well as the upper torso are now fully expelled.

28 [7198] 8:09 a.m.

The child is fully expelled.

29 [7213] 8:09 a.m.

While the surgeon holds the child by his right arm, the assistant clamps the umbilical cord in three places and cuts it through. The retractors have not yet been removed from the abdomen at this point.

30 [7217] 8:09 a.m.

Surgeon and assistant lift up the child. Now the father sitting behind a screen sees his son for the first time.

31 [7218] 8:09 a.m.

The child is presented to the clinical team and starts crying.

32 [7221] 8:09 a.m.

Straight after birth neonatal care is performed by a paediatrician. The Apgar score is ascertained to be able to roughly judge the child's health condition. During this examination the child is in a heated cot.

33 [7230] 8:10 a.m.

The placenta and part of the clamped umbilical cord are placed in an available plastic container for checking. Should the placenta not have been removed totally the mother can possibly have problems later on.

34 [7241] 8:11 a.m.

The uterus is resting on the abdominal wall, remaining amniotic fluid and blood are removed by suction. The inside of the uterus, the cavity of the uterus, is visible. Lehman states the following on this:

"Conspicuous about this method [Misgav-Ladach method of a section; Note] is that the uterus is rolled in front of the abdominal walls after expulsion of child and placenta with the argument that amniotic fluid and blood would not flow into the abdomen. Although the amniotic fluid and most of the blood definitely flowed during expulsion of the child and the placenta when the uterus was still in the abdomen. So this rolling out of the uterus [...] could [...] be forgone to shorten the operating time." (Lehmann 2006, page 232; translated English version from the original German book)

35 [7254] 8:11 a.m.

With the Green Armitage forceps the uterus is brought into the ideal position for closing up and held there.

36 [7255] 8:11 a.m.

The assistant's left index finger holds the cavity of the uterus open.

37 [7257] 8:12 a.m.

The uterus has a tear downwards. The assistant holds the tear together with the Green Armitage forceps, the surgeon stitches the tear.

38 [7372] 8:20 a.m.

The assistant holds the threads of the sutured cut in his right hand and the bottom thread of the stitched tear in his left hand. The surgeon is busy stitching further down.

39 [7384] 8:22 a.m.

The uterus is now completely sutured. The arrow shows at the bend the transition from the cut to the tear (ellipse). With this shortness of the incision further tearing of the cut in the uterus happens relatively often. This may be of importance in the case of a subsequent pregnancy (rupture of the scar).

40 [7385] 8:22 a.m.

The abdominal wall is pulled downwards with the retractors. An assistant holds the uterus up so that the surgeon can reach the bottom of the tear so as to be able to stitch it.

41 [7394] 8:23 a.m.

Suturing the uterus is now completed. The assistant starts repositioning the uterus.

42 [7395] 8:23 a.m.

The uterus is back in the abdominal cavity.

43 [7404] 8:24 a.m.

Swabs and suction apparatus are used to clean the abdominal cavity.

44 [7417] 8:25 a.m.

Minor bleeding, for example of the muscle, the edge of the fascia or the peritoneum, is stopped by electrocoagulation (heat).

45 [7418] 8:25 a.m.

Machine for coagulation (diathermy machine).

46 [7424] 8:26 a.m.

Lifting the fascia.

47 [7433] 8:28 a.m.

The fascia is closed successively.

48 [7446] 8:30 a.m.

Closing of the fascia is completed.

49 [7458] 8:32 a.m.

2 subcutaneous sutures.

50 [7472] 8:35 a.m.

Closure of the tissue completed.

51 [7479] 8:37 a.m.

Preparation of the incision for the subcuticular suture.

52 [7496] 8:40 a.m.

Running subcuticular suture performed by the surgeon.

53 [7529] 8:47 a.m.

The abdominal wall is sutured.

54 [7548] 8:51 a.m.

Used swabs are laid out on the floor and counted. This is important to make sure that none of the used swabs are inadvertently left inside the patient's abdominal cavity [cp. the report of participant 006 on page 46; Note].

55 [7555] 8:56 a.m.

The child, the patient, her husband and the surgical team have left the operating theatre.

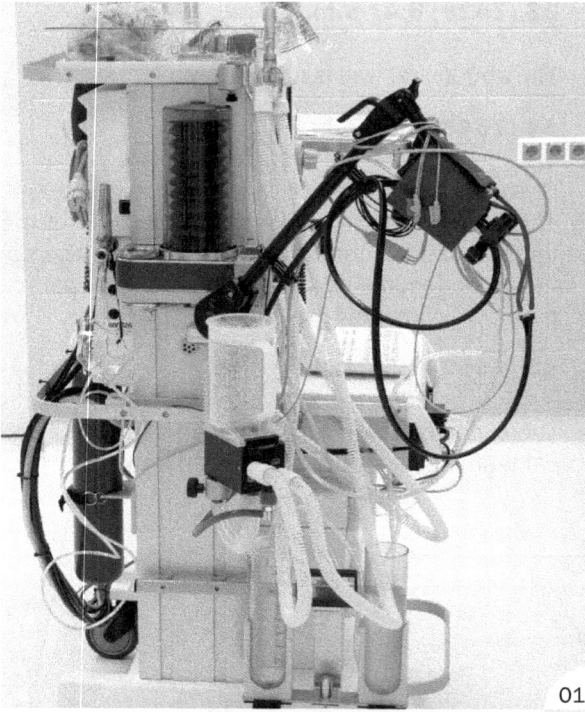
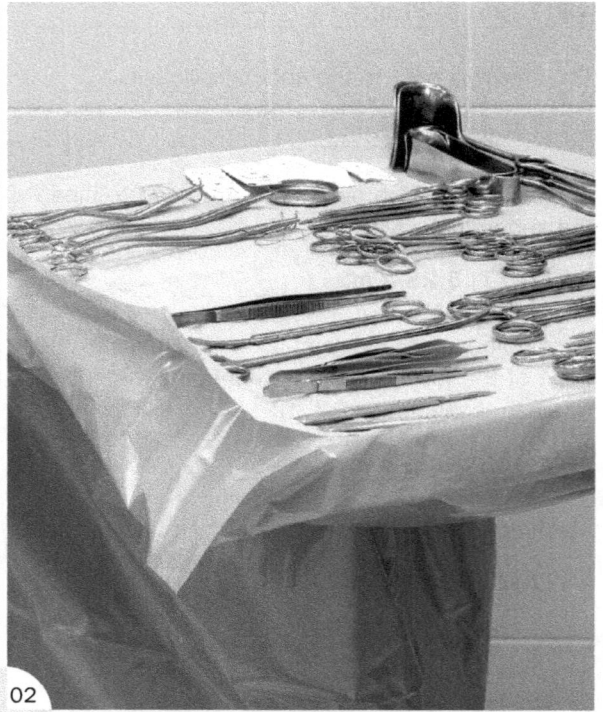

01 02
03 04

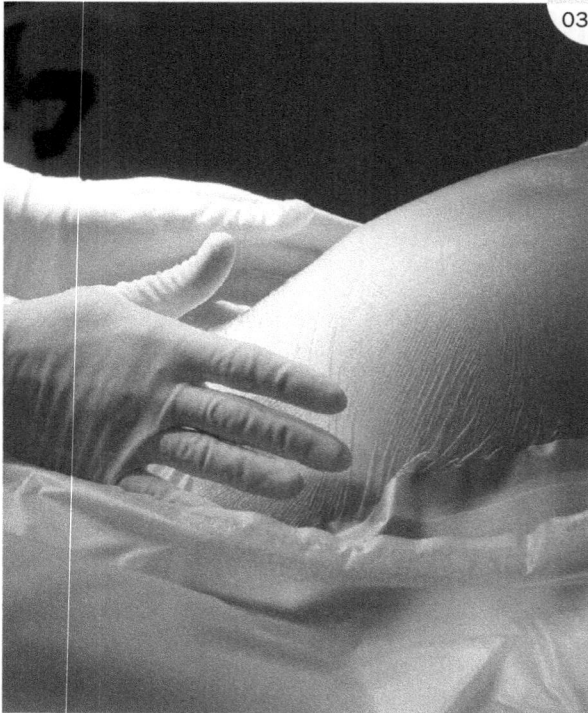
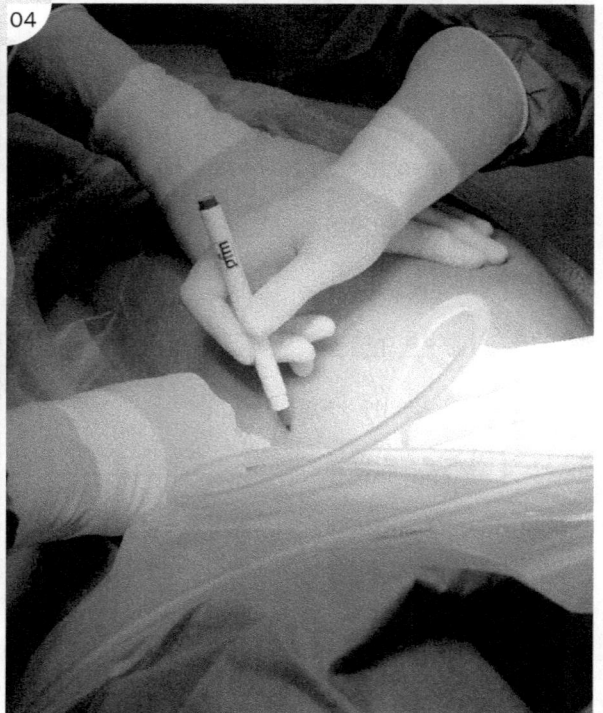

164 The "gentle Caesarean section"

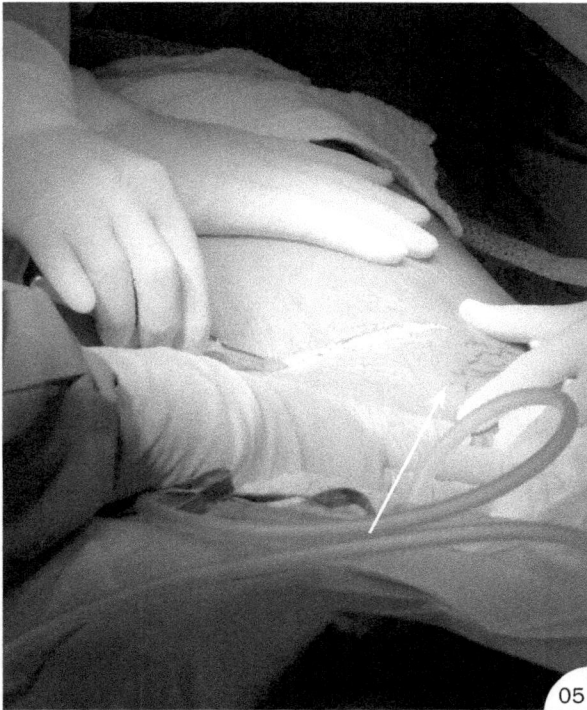 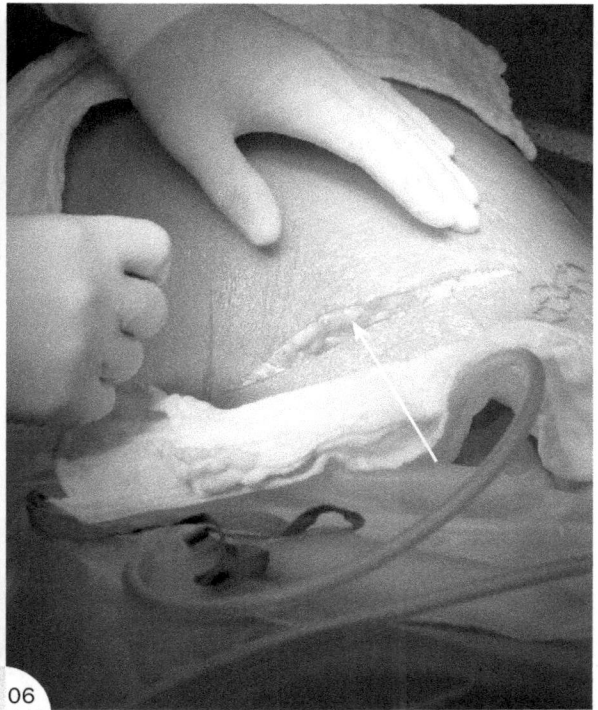

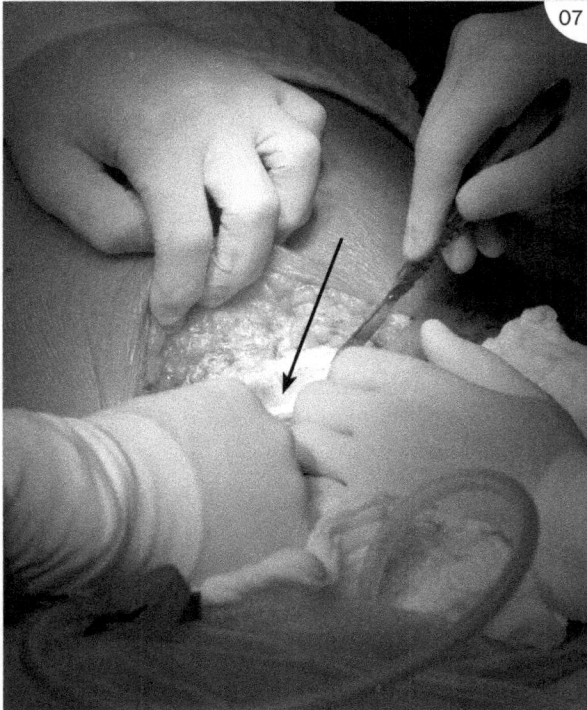 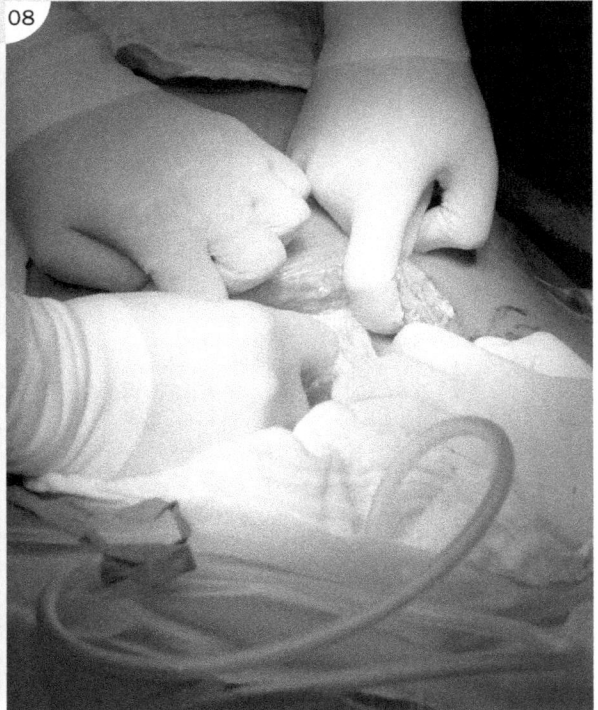

05 06
07 08

Photo report of a Caesarean section using the "Misgav Ladach" method   165

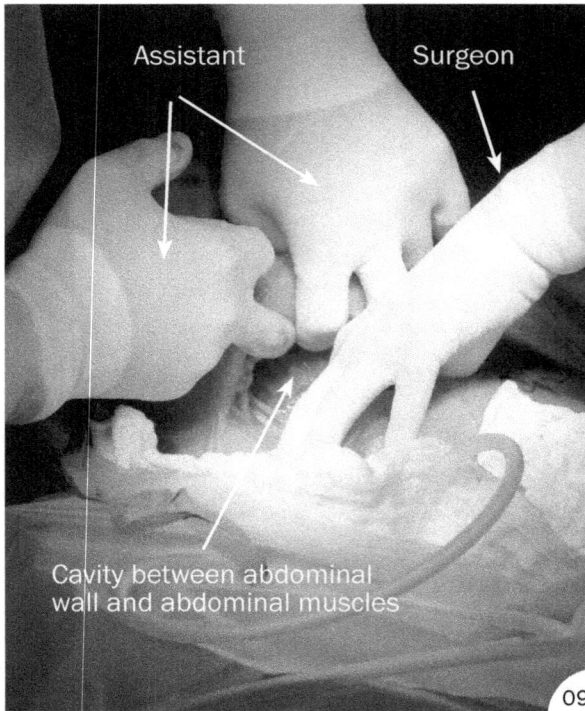

Assistant   Surgeon

Cavity between abdominal
wall and abdominal muscles

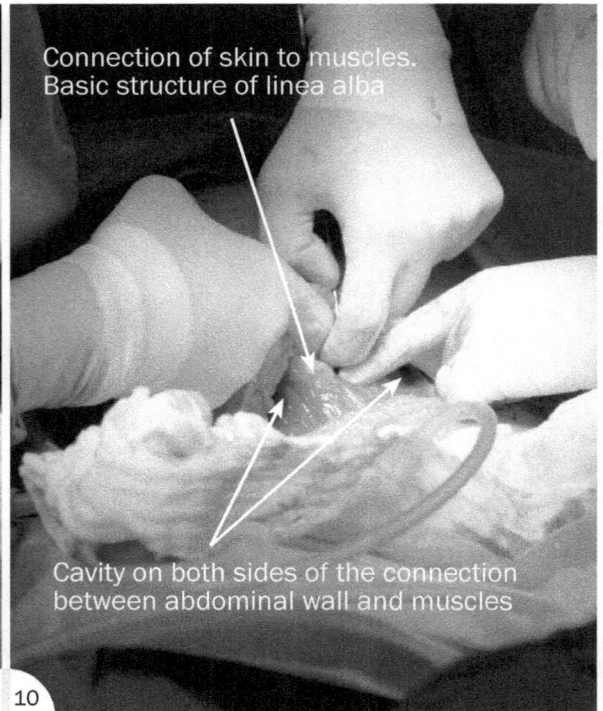

Connection of skin to muscles.
Basic structure of linea alba

Cavity on both sides of the connection
between abdominal wall and muscles

09 10
11 12

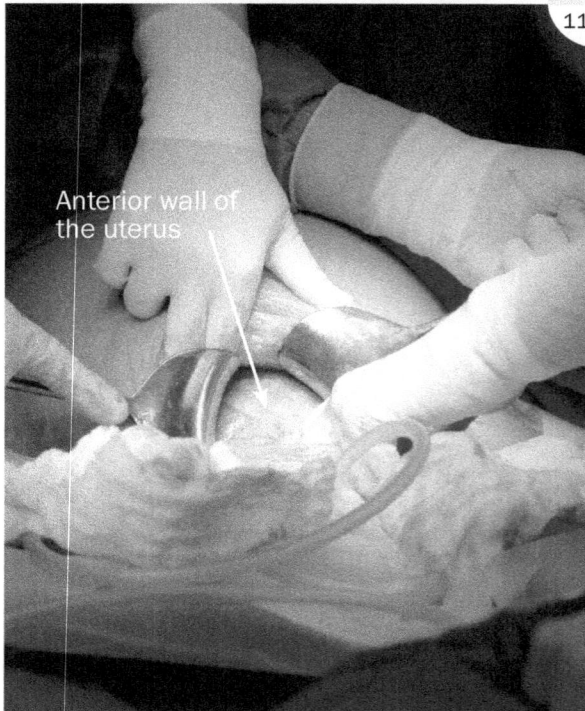

Anterior wall of
the uterus

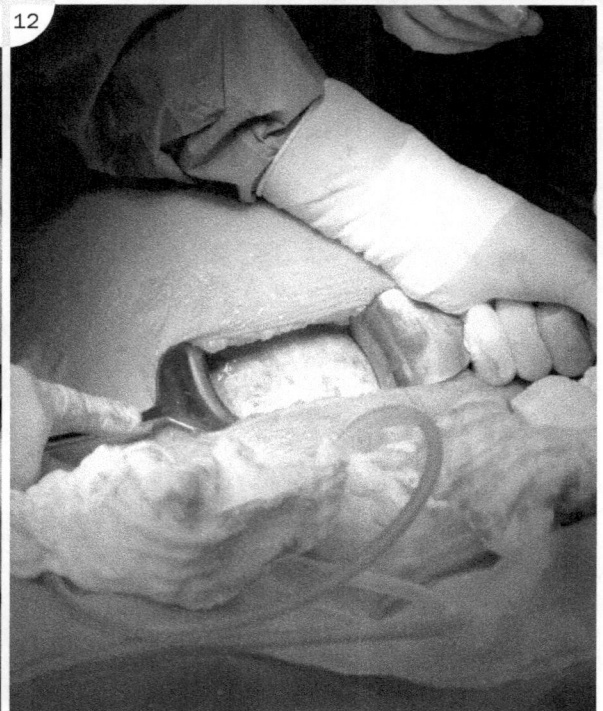

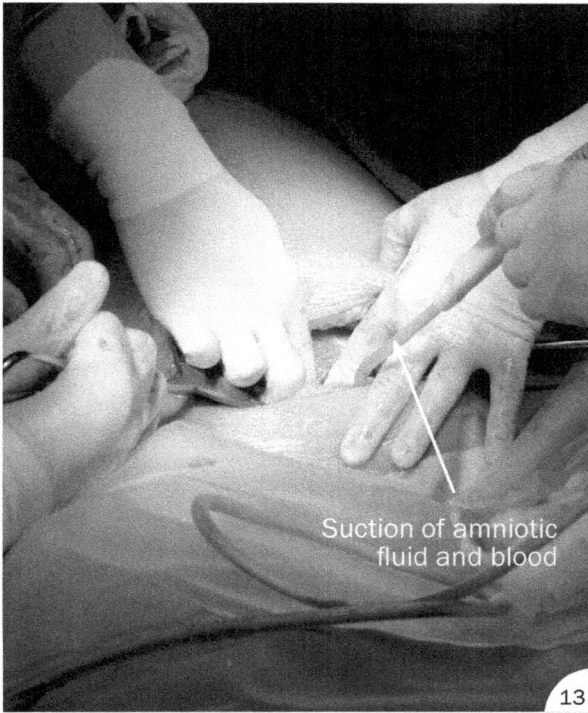
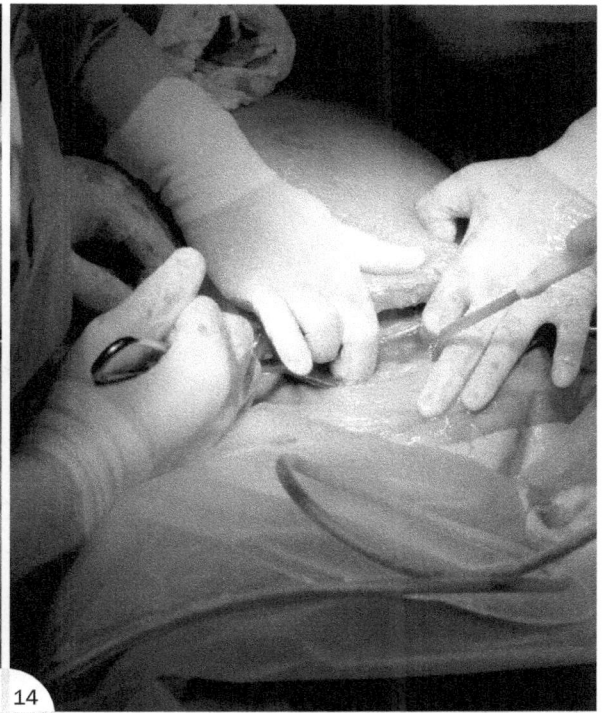
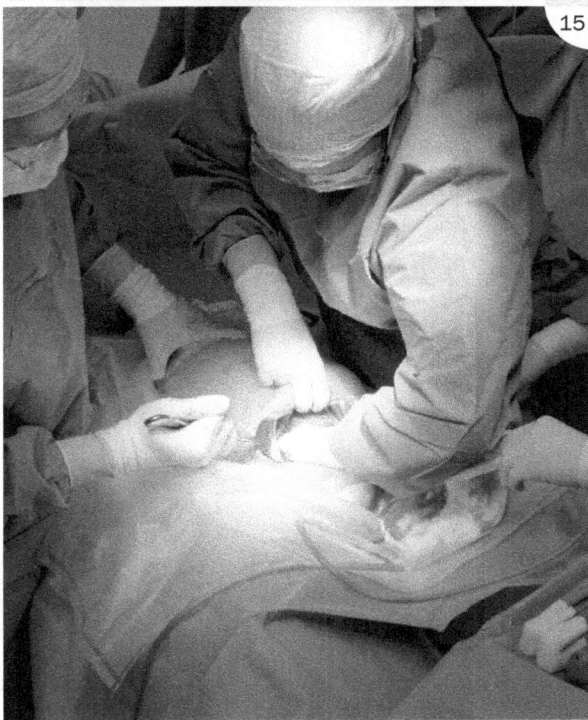
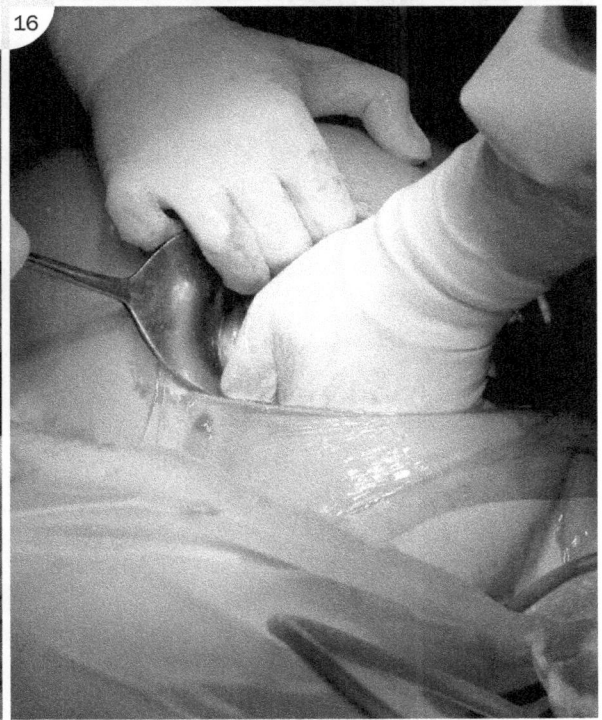

Suction of amniotic fluid and blood

Photo report of a Caesarean section using the "Misgav Ladach" method

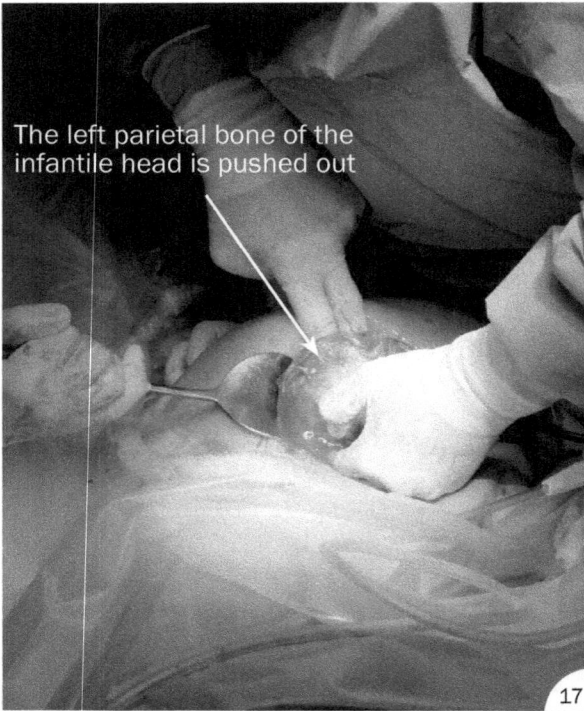

The left parietal bone of the infantile head is pushed out

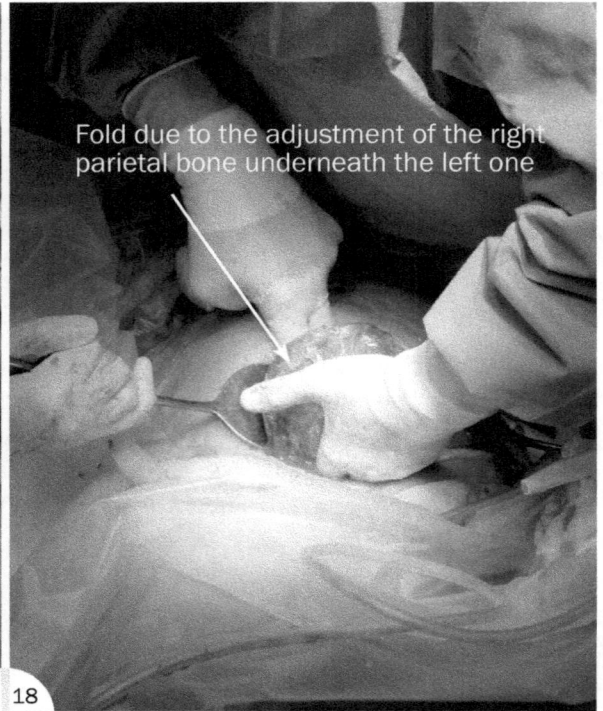

Fold due to the adjustment of the right parietal bone underneath the left one

17 18
19 20

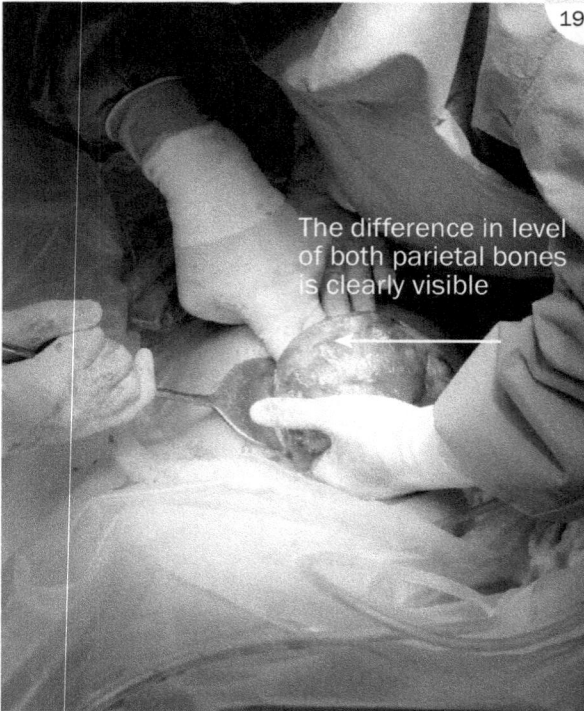

The difference in level of both parietal bones is clearly visible

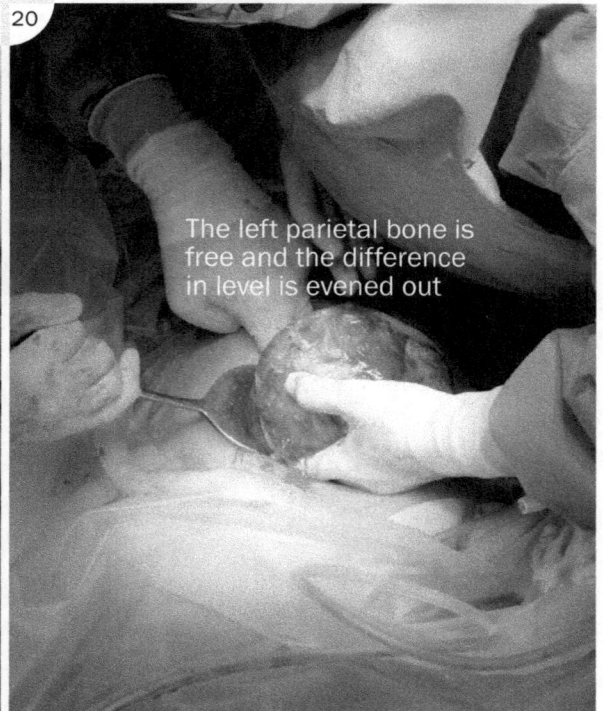

The left parietal bone is free and the difference in level is evened out

The "gentle Caesarean section"

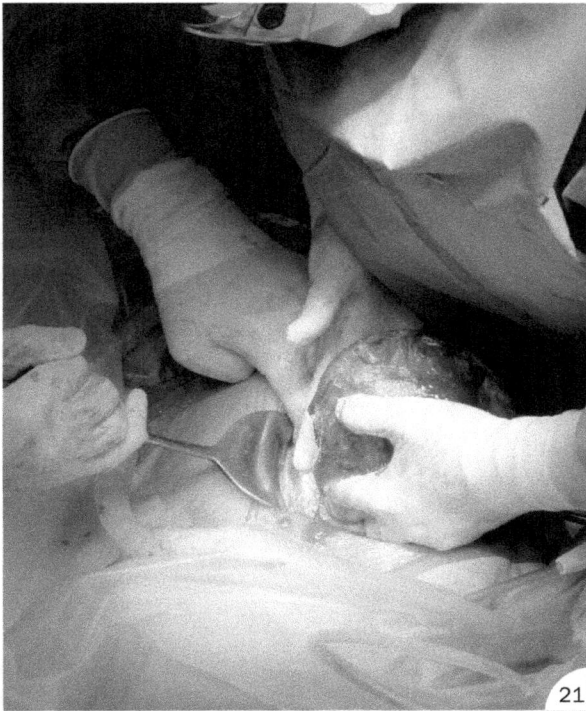

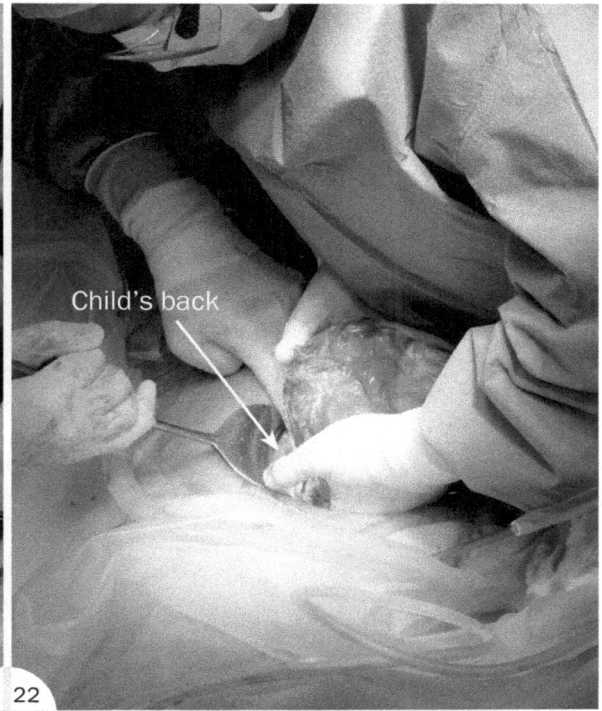
Child's back

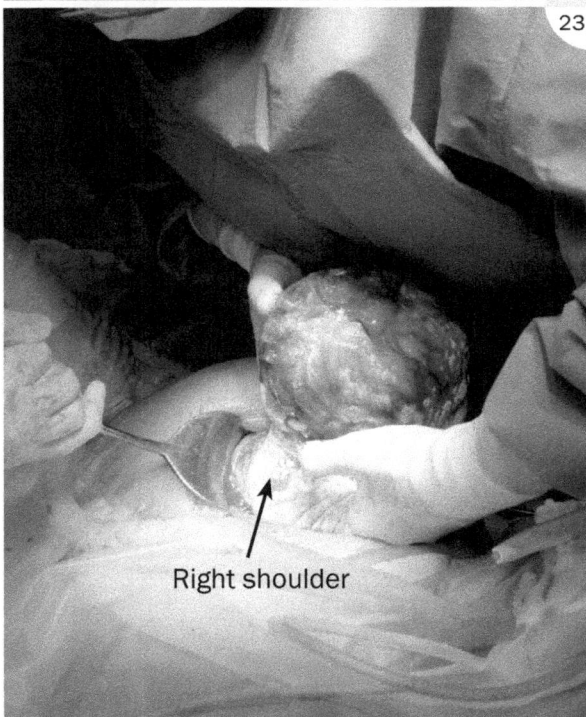
Right shoulder

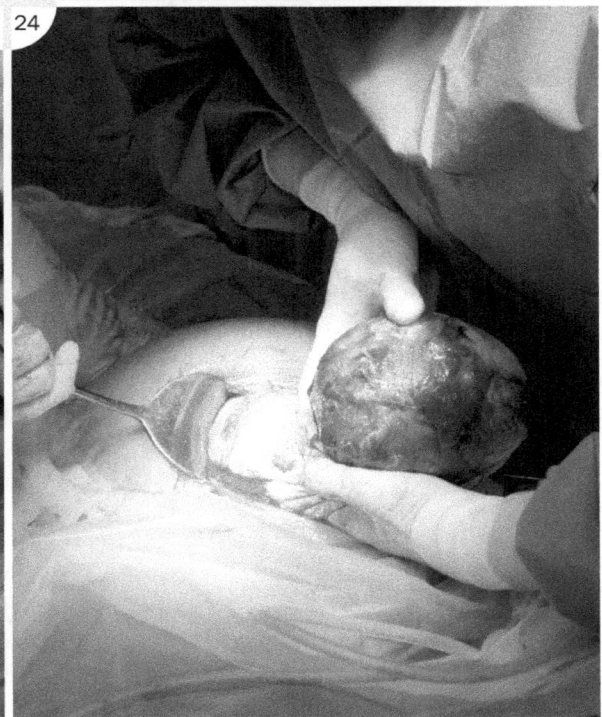

Photo report of a Caesarean section using the "Misgav Ladach" method

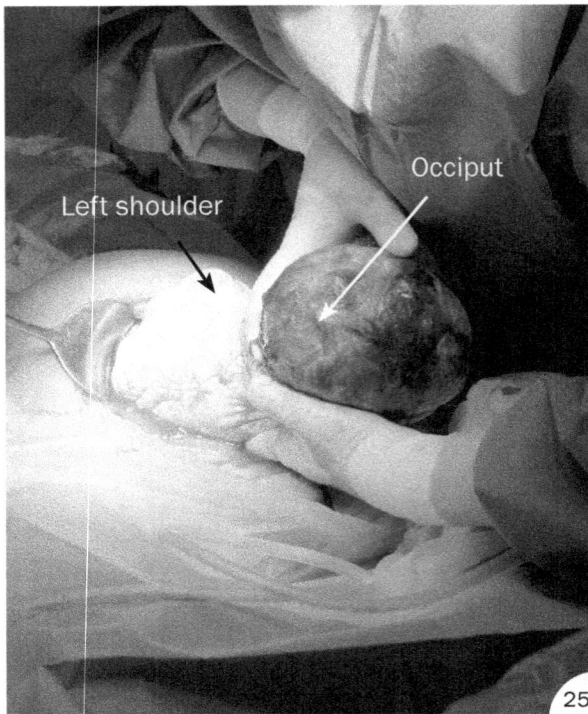

Left shoulder

Occiput

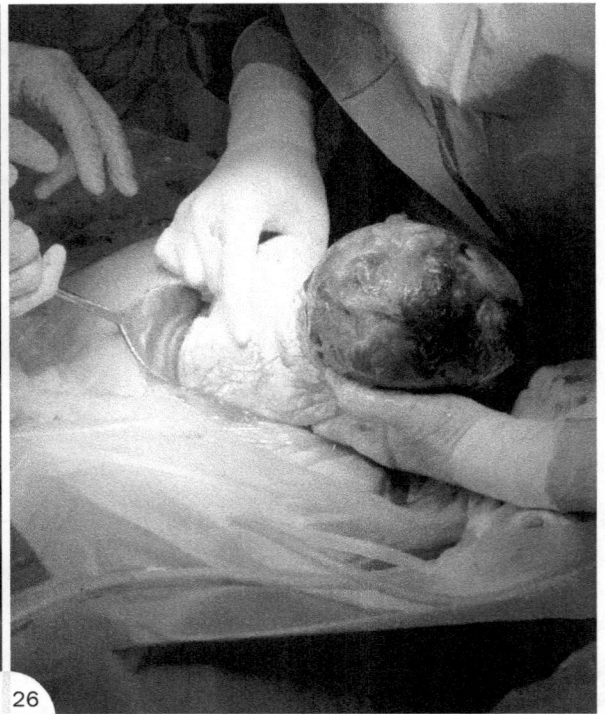

25 26
27 28

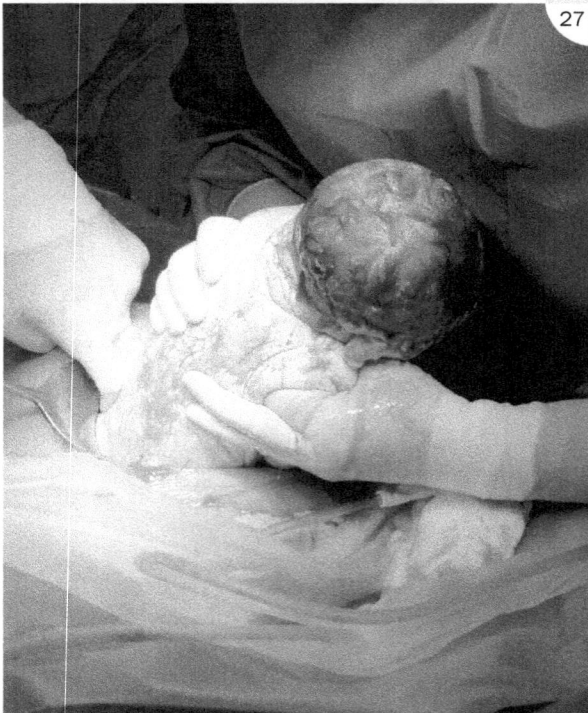

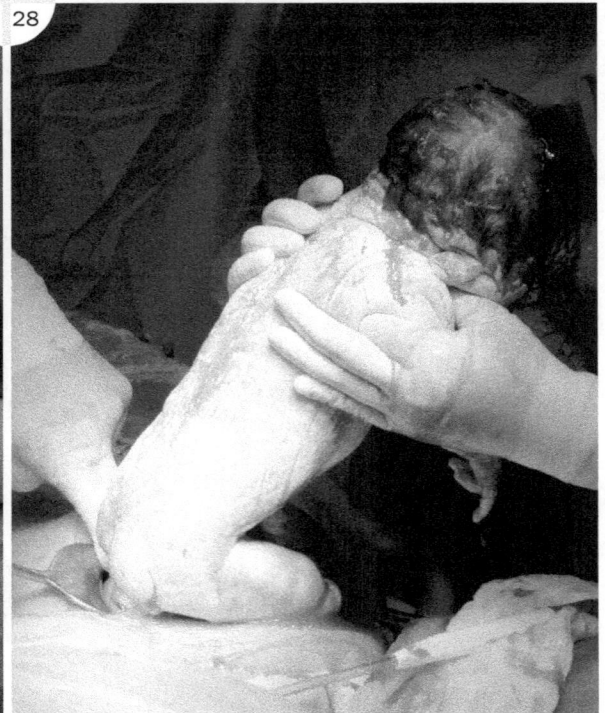

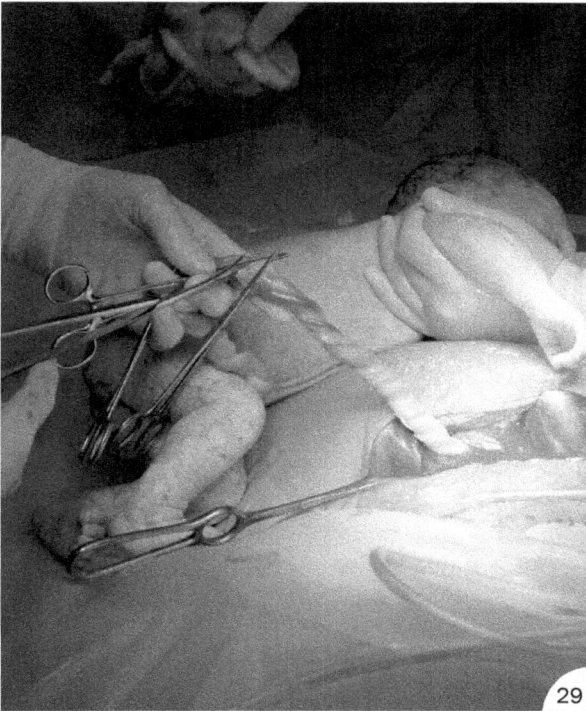

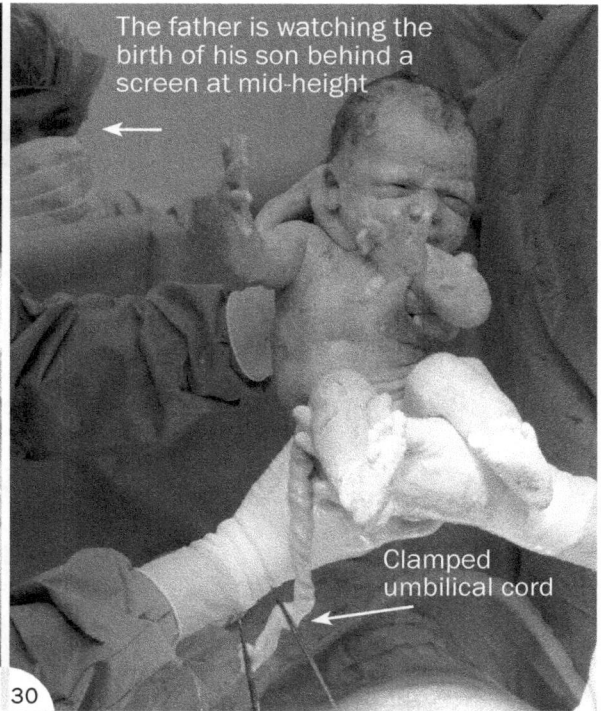

The father is watching the birth of his son behind a screen at mid-height

Clamped umbilical cord

29 30
31 32

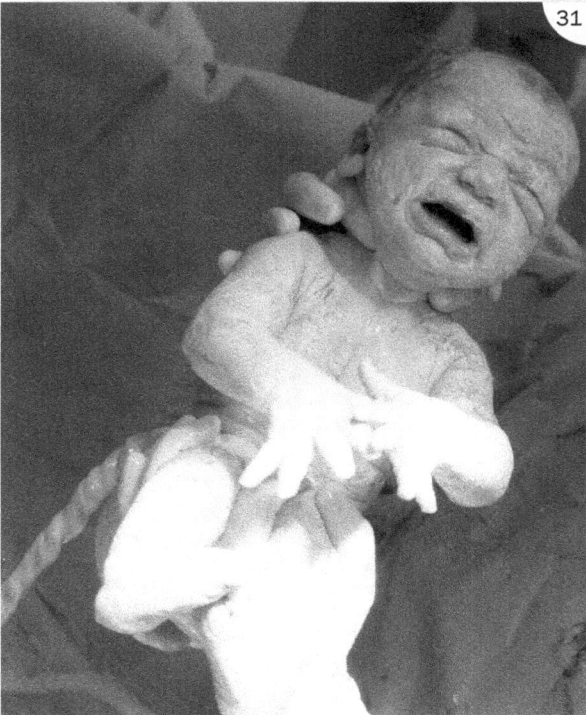

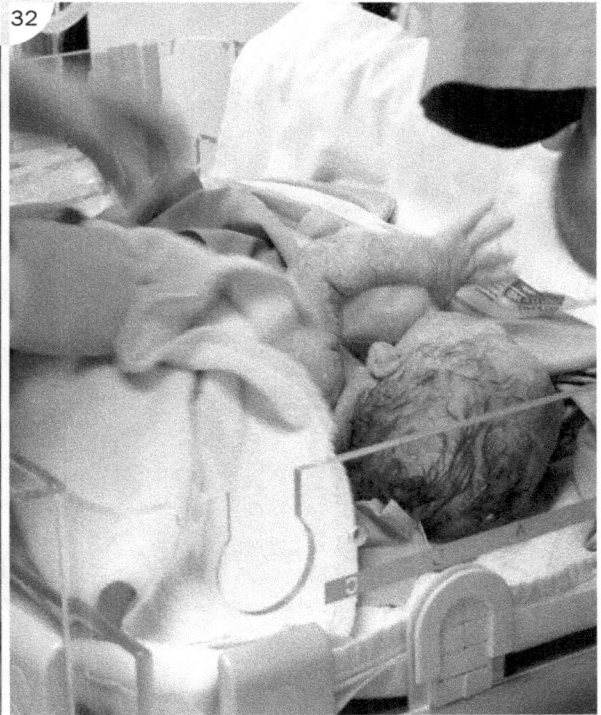

Photo report of a Caesarean section using the "Misgav Ladach" method

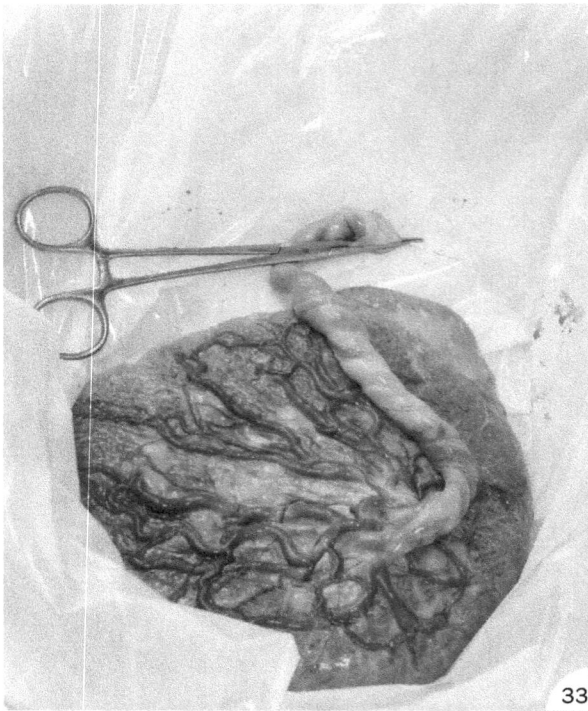
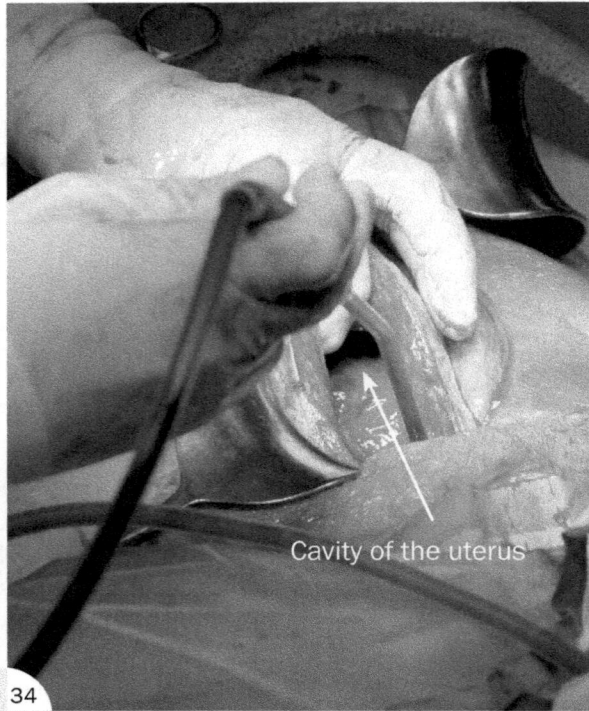

Cavity of the uterus

33 34
35 36

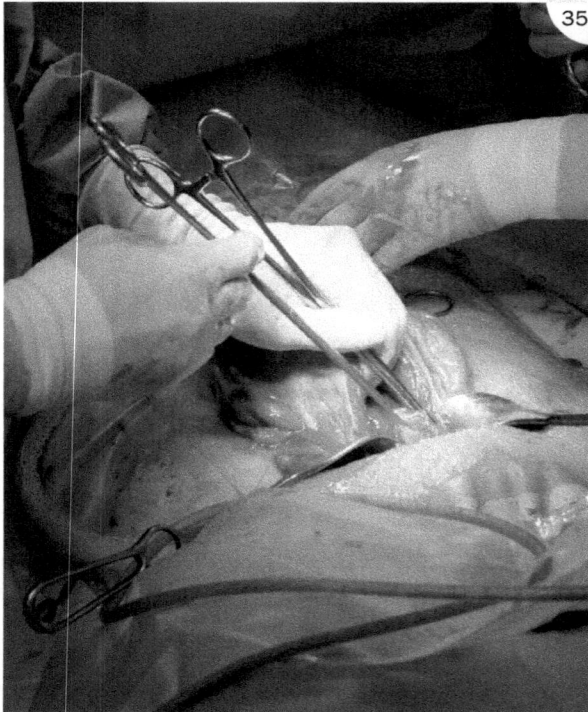
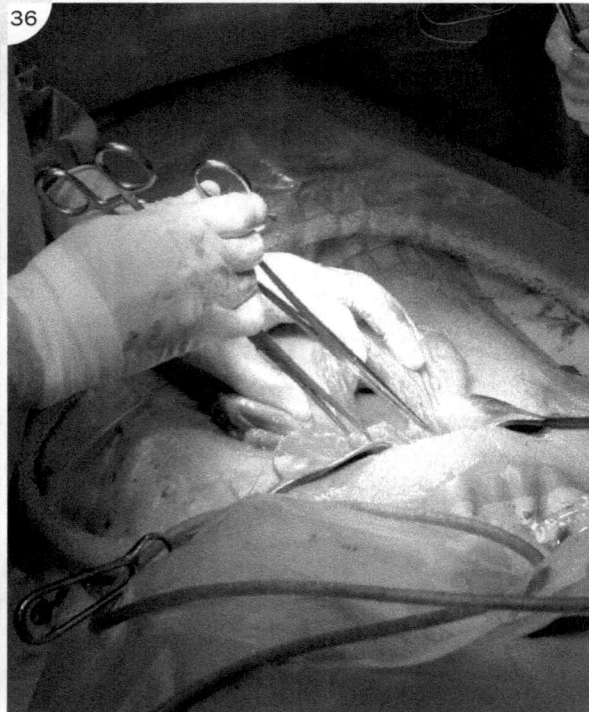

The "gentle Caesarean section"

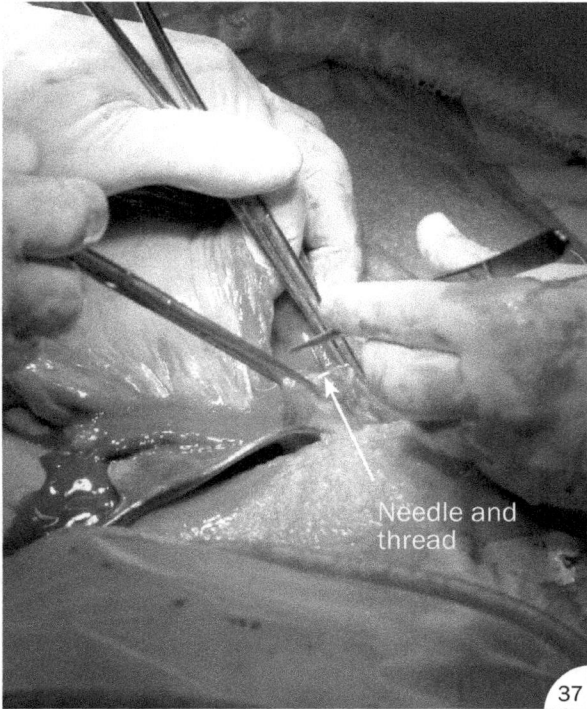

Needle and thread

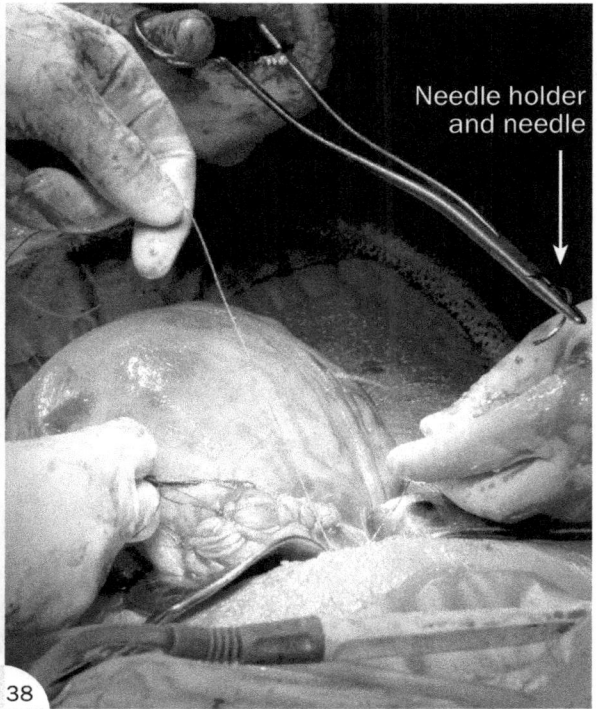

Needle holder and needle

37 38
39 40

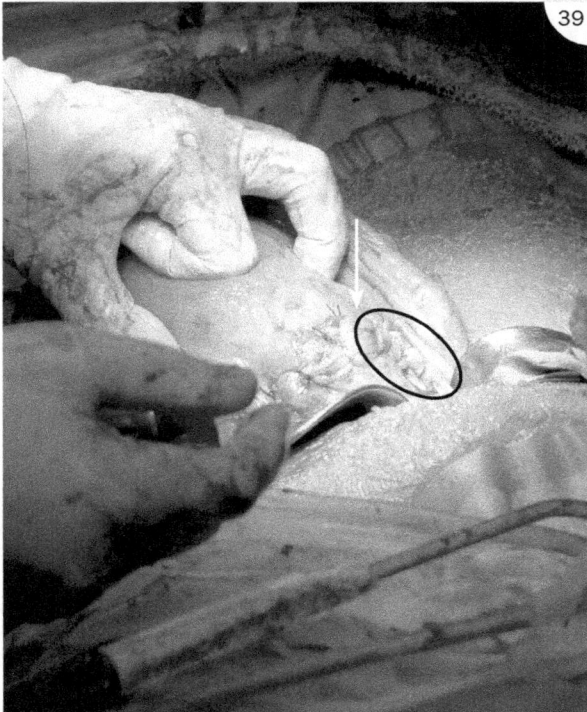

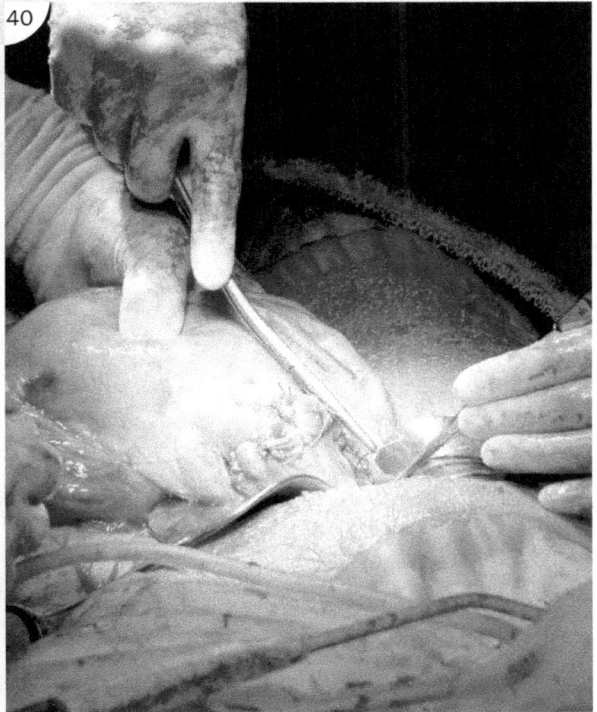

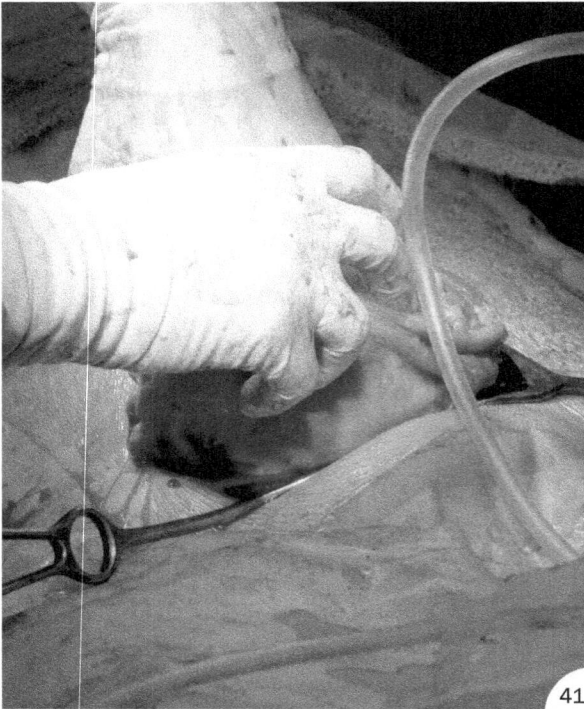
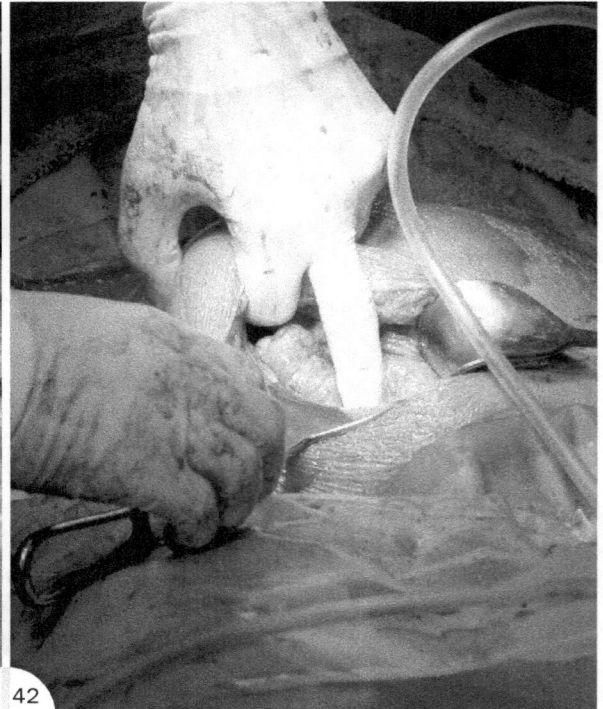
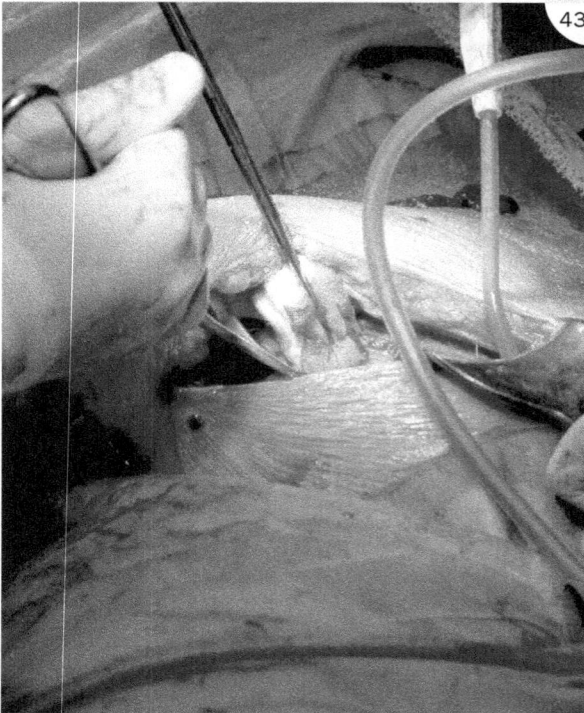
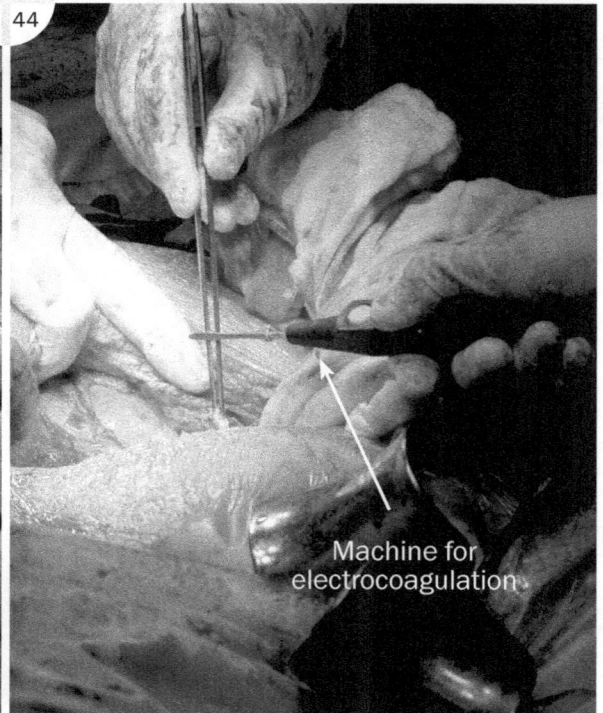

Machine for electrocoagulation

The "gentle Caesarean section"

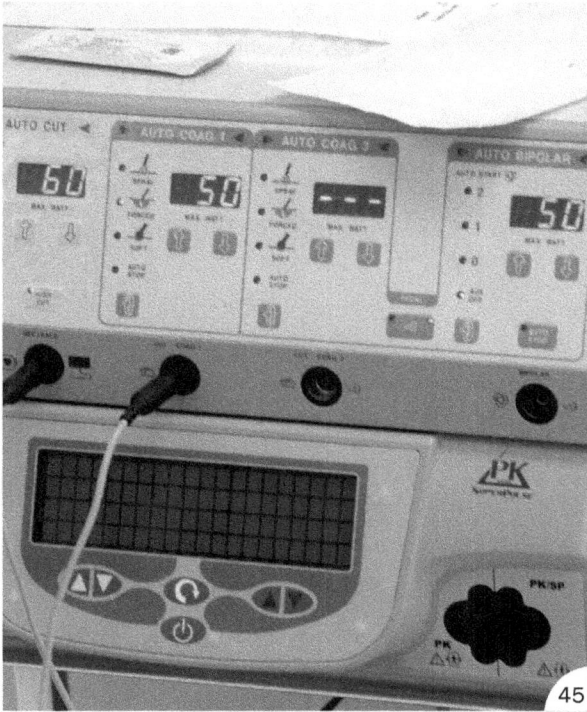

45 46
47 48

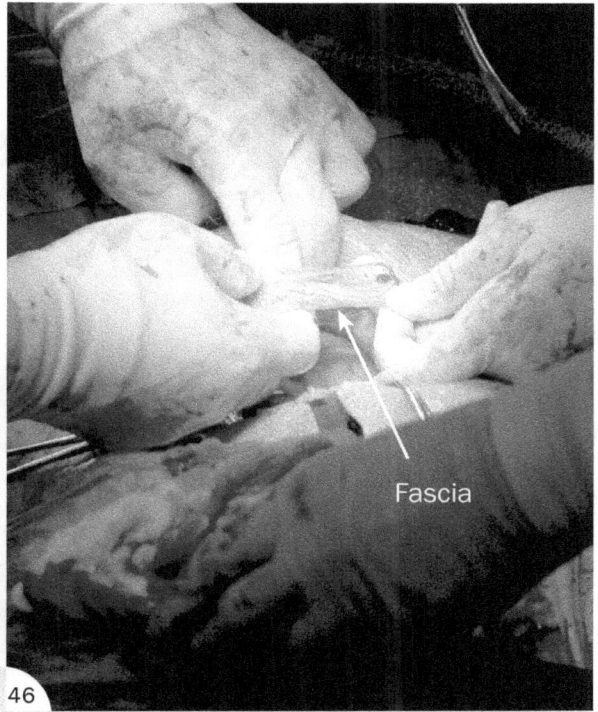

Fascia

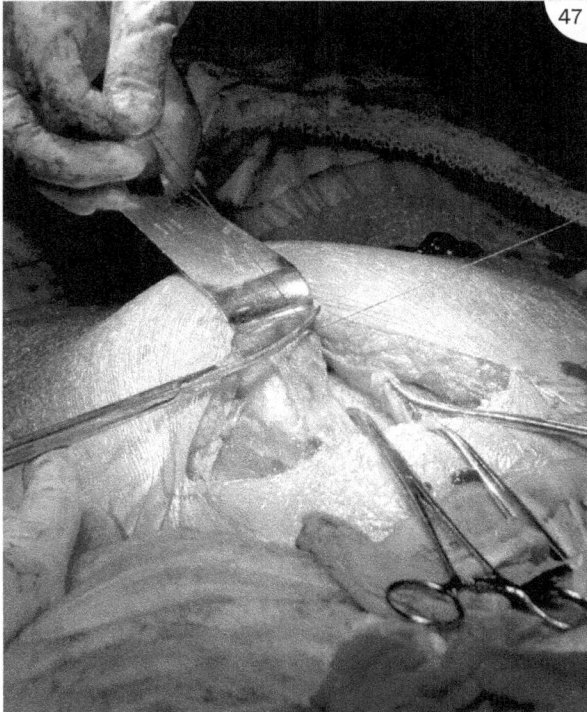

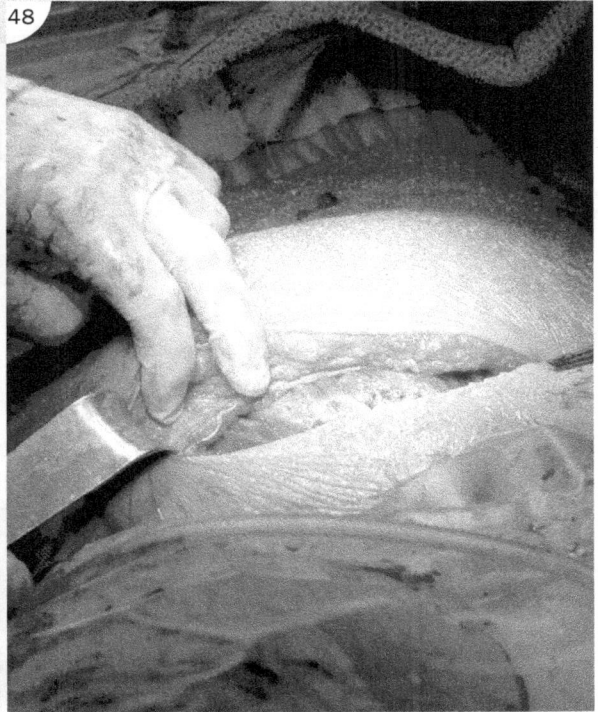

Photo report of a Caesarean section using the "Misgav Ladach" method   175

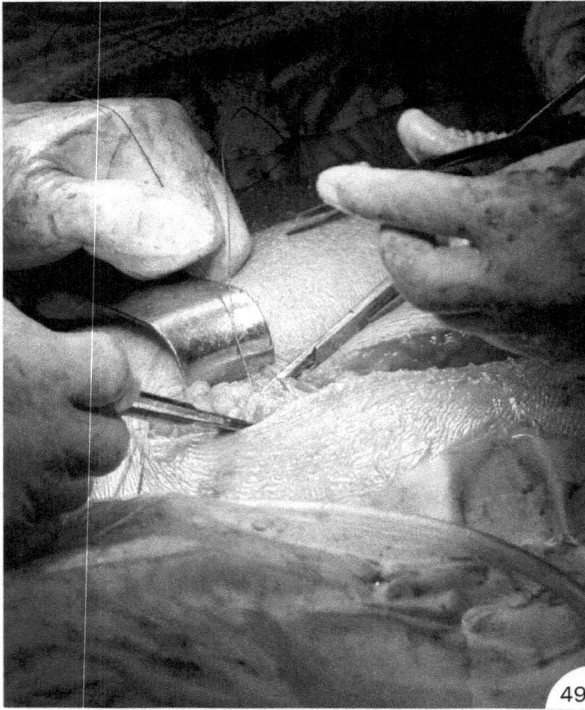
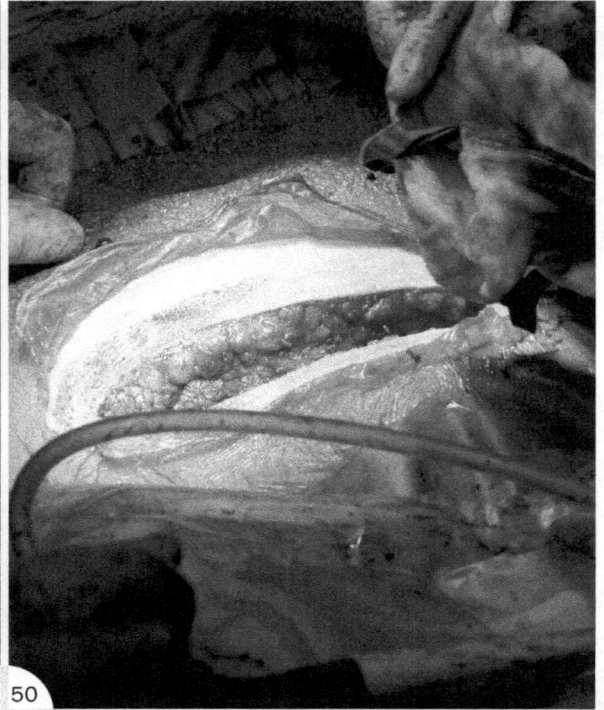
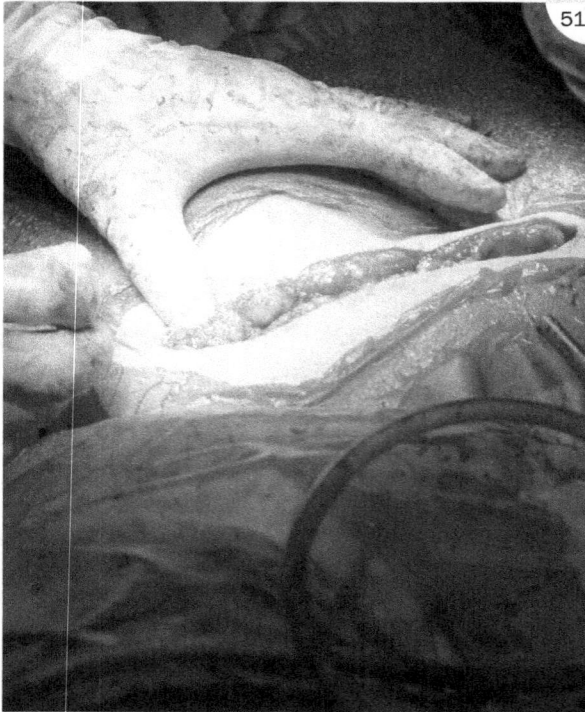
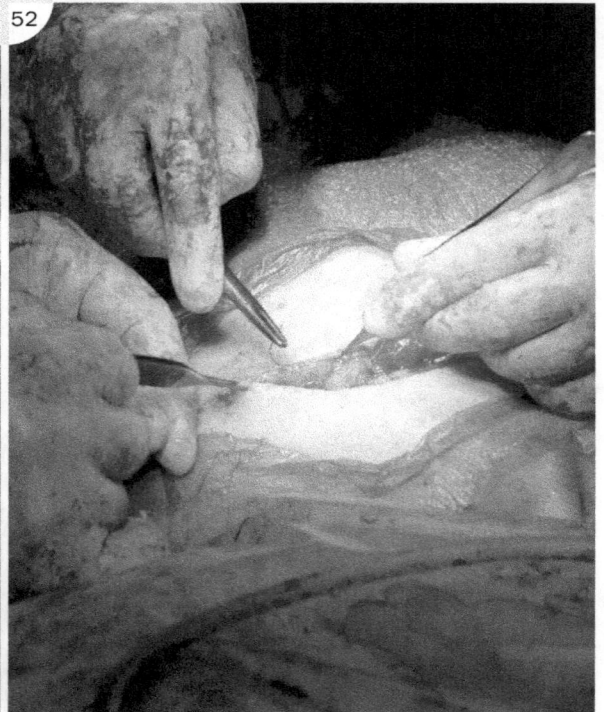

49 50
51 52

The "gentle Caesarean section"

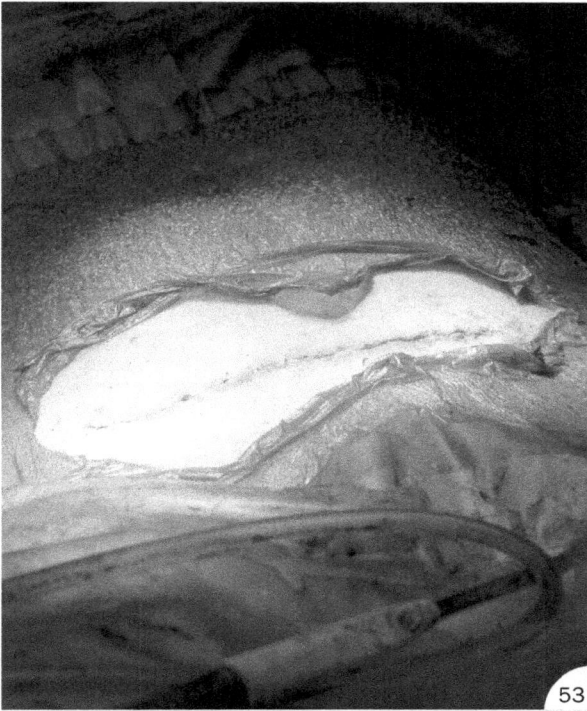
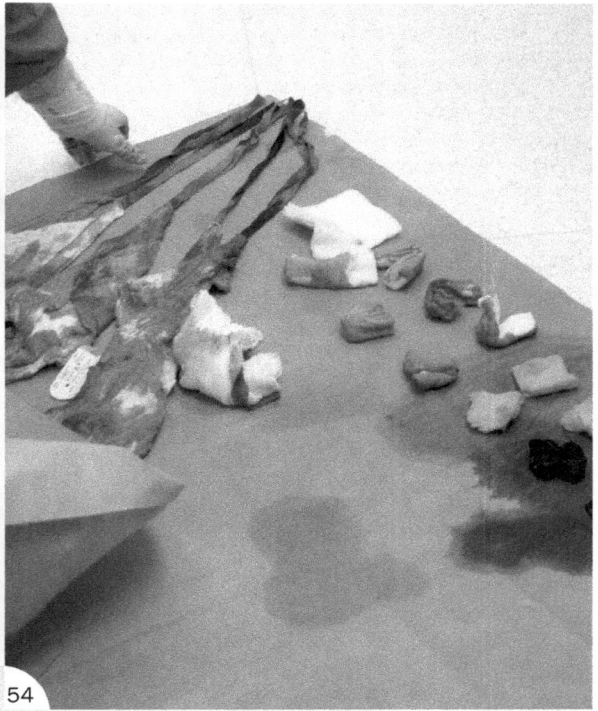
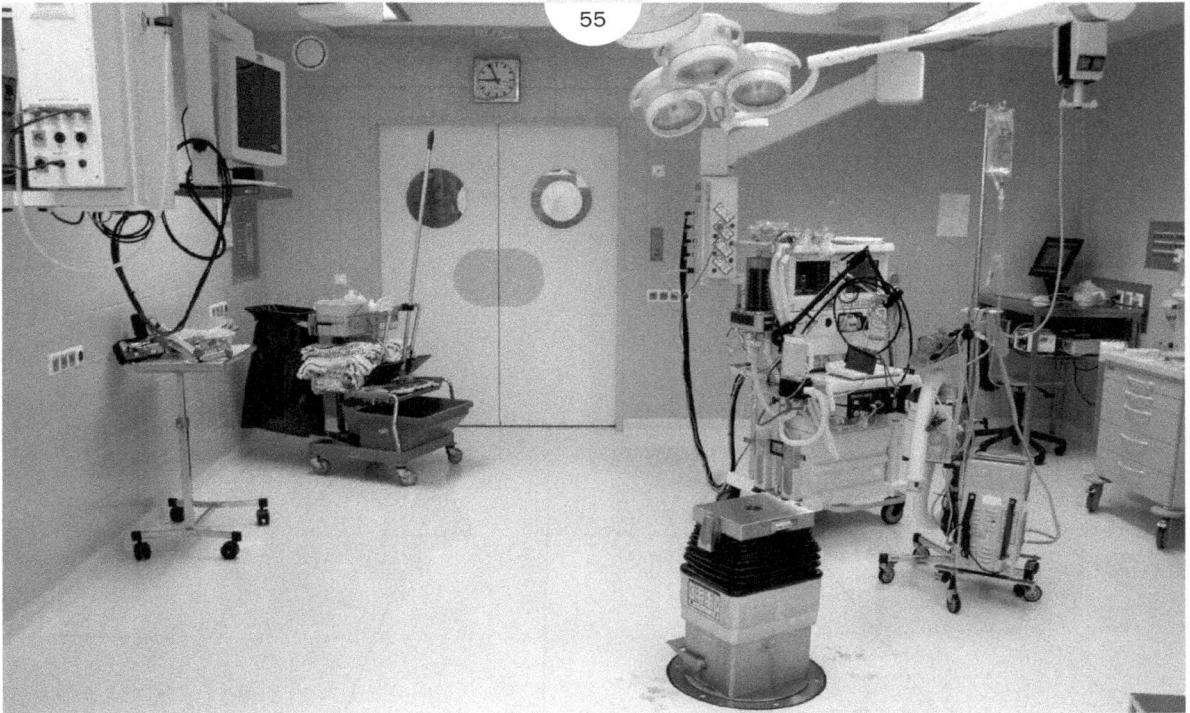

Photo report of a Caesarean section using the "Misgav Ladach" method

After gaining insight a quick overview:

Possible conclusions

Someone approaches you and says: "We are going to cut open your abdomen now." You ask: "Why?" The answer is: "Because it is easier to schedule, because we are afraid you might sue us and because you yourself want it!"

This or something like this could be a nightmare. The nightmare of a Caesarean section.

For many mothers being cut open as a living being means humiliation and powerlessness. They do not see the obstetric surgery as procedure they have chosen for themselves but mostly feel deprived of their right to experience birth. They feel wounded – physically and mentally.

And as if that were not enough. Many women need the Caesarean section – whatever the reason may be – and have to let a lot of strangers care for them during the birth of their child.

It is not about preventing the Caesarean section at any cost but about allowing the surgery to be as natural as possible in case of an emergency.

A woman who is confronted with the birth of a child for the first time in her life will hardly be able to express her wishes concerning the procedure of the surgery should a Caesarean section be necessary. At best she will know about the performance of the surgery from friends' narratives. Maybe she has seen a report on television or has read about it in a magazine. Possibly she also read this book and was, thereby, able to increase her knowledge.

However, what the Caesarean section really means every woman will only be able to answer for herself a lot later.

Caesarean surgery: Preparation, procedure, aftercare

Our survey on Caesareans has shown that women often remember certain details, which may have seemed to be irrelevant, years later. Evidently the way they were treated prior to, during and after the surgery for example becomes more important with time.

However, memories of the Caesarean surgery need not be unpleasant, as many of our Caesarean mothers demonstrate.

In collaboration with midwives and obstetricians we have worked out a few points, which are important from our point of view, to allow Caesarean surgery to be as natural as possible in case it is really indispensible.

Heeding these "recommendations" – which we shaped using the thoughts of obstetricians – should contribute to a transition, as gently as possible, from pregnancy to motherhood. When surgery is necessary the newborn in particular should, where possible, have a gentle and not abrupt beginning to life outside the womb.

Recommendations for Caesarean births (Version March 2009)

1. Check the indication

- Second opinion — Is the Caesarean section really inevitable? Get a second opinion if necessary (midwife, obstetrician, physician – depending on the indication).

2. If medically possible: Time for birth set at the mother and child's pace

- Scheduled section — Many midwives say that it would be ideal to wait for natural contractions. Sometimes even the obstetricians in charge agree. Alternatively, if possible, 3 hours prior to the section put the pregnant woman on a drip to bring on contractions so that the uterus and the baby can prepare for the surgical intervention.
- Support — The partner, a familiar midwife or another confidant can convey the mother's wishes when she is too weak or unresponsive. Organising this before the scheduled section should not be forgotten.

3. Preparing for the surgery

- What is going to happen? — Detailed, comprehensible explanation for mother (and partner) of what is going to happen – especially in the case of an emergency Caesarean section!
- Anaesthesia — If possible avoid general anaesthesia. With epidural/spinal anaesthesia: do not let the mother fall asleep unnecessarily after the child is removed from the uterus because the important first contact is lost thereby.

4. During the surgery

- What is going to happen? — Detailed, comprehensible explanation for mother (and partner) of what is happening at the moment.
- Cord clamping — For medical reasons (massive loss of blood) it is not safe to wait for the umbilical cord to stop pulsating with a Caesarean section. To alleviate possible imbalances or disorders the child has, due to the immediate cutting of the cord, it might be possible to use craniosacral therapy or osteopathy about 2 weeks after the Caesarean section
- Vaccination — Vaccinating the infant with "vaginal flora" of the healthy and well nourished mother may possibly be conducive to the normal colonisation of the infant's intestine.
- Stem cells — Do the parents want stem cells to be withdrawn?
- Suction — If medically possible no suctioning of the baby's nose because this causes the mucous membranes to swell and the child who breathes solely through his or her nose is distressed. Intensive manipulation occurs when suctioning the baby's palate. This irritates the suck reflex and can result in difficulties with breastfeeding.
- First contact — Baby and mother are allowed to get to know each other right after birth, skin on skin, not wrapped in sheets. Have a warm blanket ready. Bathing and dressing the child take place later.
- Breastfeeding — Latching for the first time in the operating theatre, if possible. The mother is supported by the midwife/nurse in getting the baby latched on properly.
- Paediatrician — Wait for bonding and the first breastfeed. Neonatal status only after breastfeeding.

5. After birth

- Umbilical cord/placenta — Show and explain. Make it possible for the mother to take both home with her when discharged from the hospital if she wishes to do so.
- Postnatal period — Constant support of the Caesarean mother (breastfeeding, getting up, caring for the child, ...). Mobilising of the mother and treatment of the Caesarean scar by the midwife/therapist.
- Surgery report — Issue and automatic delivery of an informative surgery report on discharge.

From: C-Section Moms by Caroline Oblasser • www.editionriedenburg.at

Appendix

Questionnaire for Caesarean mothers

Questionnaire for obstetric experts

My personal Caesarean questionnaire

Questionnaire for Caesarean mothers:

Questions with a check box were to be marked with a cross, for questions to be answered freely an extra sheet of lined paper was available. Original format DIN A4.

All data will be made anonymous before publication, kept in confidence and not forwarded to a third party!

1.) Statistical personal data.

1.1) Surname / Given name _____ 1.2) Title _____

1.3) Date of birth: _____ . _____ . 19_____ 1.4) Time _____ : _____

1.5) I was delivered by Caesarean section myself. yes ☐ no ☐

1.6) My mother was delivered by Caesarean section. yes ☐ no ☐

1.7) I have given birth to a total of _____ child(ren) and had _____ Caesarean section(s).

1.8) My marital status: single ☐ living with a partner ☐ married ☐

widowed ☐ divorced ☐ other ☐: _____

1.9) Education compulsory education ☐ apprenticeship ☐ vocational school ☐

A-levels ☐ academic studies ☐ other ☐: _____

1.10) Occupation _____

2.) When I hear the word "Caesarean section" the following 5 words come to mind spontaneously:

2.1) 1. _____

2.2) 2. _____

2.3) 3. _____

2.4) 4. _____

2.5) 5. _____

My
1st child

3.1) Date of birth: _____ . _____ . _____   3.2) Time _____ : _____

3.3) Sex: girl ☐   boy ☐   3.4) Caesarean birth?   yes ☐   no ☐

3.5) Short comment about the birth of my 1st child

_____

_____

My
2nd child

3.1) Date of birth: _____ . _____ . _____   3.2) Time _____ : _____

3.3) Sex: girl ☐   boy ☐   3.4) Caesarean birth?   yes ☐   no ☐

3.5) Short comment about the birth of my 2nd child

_____

_____

My
3rd child

3.1) Date of birth: _____ . _____ . _____   3.2) Time _____ : _____

3.3) Sex: girl ☐   boy ☐   3.4) Caesarean birth?   yes ☐   no ☐

3.5) Short comment about the birth of my 3rd child

_____

_____

My
4th child

3.1) Date of birth: _____ . _____ . _____   3.2) Time _____ : _____

3.3) Sex: girl ☐   boy ☐   3.4) Caesarean birth?   yes ☐   no ☐

3.5) Short comment about the birth of my 4th child

_____

_____

My
5th child

3.1) Date of birth: _____ . _____ . _____   3.2) Time _____ : _____

3.3) Sex: girl ☐   boy ☐   3.4) Caesarean birth?   yes ☐   no ☐

3.5) Short comment about the birth of my 5th child

_____

_____

4.) My Caesarean child(ren).

Please complete one sheet, for the questions under point 4.), for each of your Caesarean children (also for multiples). For multiples please supply identical information using one sheet only.

4.1a)   My   1ˢᵗ ☐   2ⁿᵈ ☐   3ʳᵈ ☐   4ᵗʰ ☐   5ᵗʰ ☐   child delivered by Caesarean section.

4.1b)   Child's date of birth _____ . _____ . _____   4.2) Time _____ : _____

4.3a)   Sex: girl ☐   boy ☐   4.3b) single ☐   multiple ☐, namely: _____

4.3c)   Head circumference: _____ cm   4.3d) Height: _____ cm   4.3e) Weight: _____ g

4.4)   Duration of pregnancy: _____ weeks of pregnancy

4.5)   The cost of the birth was paid privately / a private supplementary health insurance was used.
yes ☐   no ☐

4.6)   The Caesarean section was   planned ☐   not planned ☐

4.7)   The Caesarean section was an emergency section ☐   an elective section ☐   neither of these ☐

4.8)   The decision for the Caesarean section was made during birth.   yes ☐   no ☐

4.9)   Who decided on the Caesarean in the end? (multiple answers possible)
physician ☐   midwife ☐   myself ☐   other ☐: _____

4.10)   My partner was present during the Caesarean and stood by me: yes ☐   no ☐

4.11)   Reason for the Caesarean section (indication, e.g. breech presentation) was the following:
_____

4.12)   Prior to the Caesarean, I had real (natural) contractions.
yes ☐, duration approx. _____ hours   no ☐

4.13)   Prior to the Caesarean, I had artificial / induced contractions brought on by drugs.
yes ☐, duration approx. _____ hours   no ☐

4.14)   Prior to the Caesarean, I received drugs.   no ☐   yes ☐, to my knowledge:
_____

4.15)   The Caesarean was performed under the following anaesthesia: spinal anaesthesia ☐
epidural anaesthesia ☐   general anaesthesia ☐   other ☐: _____

4.16)   The Caesarean proceeded without complications
yes ☐   no ☐, following complications occurred:
_____
_____

4.17)   I wanted to breastfeed after birth.   yes ☐   no ☐

4.18)   I was able to breastfeed without difficulty after the Caesarean.
yes ☐   no ☐, following complications occurred:
_____

4.19)   Breastfeeding duration:
0-6 months ☐   6-12 months ☐   more than 1 year ☐
more than 2 years ☐   I am still breastfeeding ☐   I never breastfed ☐

4.) My Caesarean child(ren). (Continued)

Please complete one sheet, for the questions under point 4.), for each of your Caesarean children (also for multiples).
For multiples please supply identical information using one sheet only.

4.20)   The very first (eye-)contact with my child took place

during the operation ☐   approx. _____ hours after the operation ☐

4.21)   The first intensive physical contact with my child took place

during the operation ☐   approx. _____ hours after the operation ☐

4.22)   I find that the Caesarean interfered with the mother-child bonding.

no ☐   yes ☐, namely as follows:

_____

_____

4.23)   I would have preferred a natural (vaginal) birth.   yes ☐   no ☐

4.24a) I was afraid of pain during birth.   yes ☐   no ☐

4.24b) I was afraid of perineal trauma.   yes ☐   no ☐

4.25)   I was afraid of a possible Caesarean section.   yes ☐   no ☐

4.26)   The possibility of a Caesarean was prognosticated.   yes ☐   no ☐

4.27)   I miss having a natural birth experience.   yes ☐   no ☐

4.28)   I feel inferior due to having missed out on the experience of birth.   yes ☐   no ☐

4.29)   I experienced the Caesarean section as traumatic.   yes ☐   no ☐

4.30)   The Caesarean gives me the feeling of not having done everything for my child.   yes ☐   no ☐

4.31)   I suffered from depression after the Caesarean.
        no ☐   yes ☐, namely

_____

4.32)   My child was injured during/through the Caesarean section.
        no ☐   yes ☐, namely

_____

4.33)   My child had serious/extreme health problems (e.g. also asthma, allergies, …).
        no ☐   yes ☐, namely

_____

4.34)   My child has health problems now.
        no ☐   yes ☐, namely

_____

4.35)   I noticed peculiarities in my child, which I ascribe to the Caesarean birth.
        no ☐   yes ☐, namely

_____

5.1)   I had health problems after or I have been having health problems since my Caesarean section(s).
       no ☐   yes ☐, namely

_____

5.2)   My Caesarean scar(s) healed without a problem.   no ☐   yes ☐, namely

_____

5.3)   I can feel my Caesarean scar(s).   no ☐   yes ☐, namely

_____

5.4)   I took care of / treated my Caesarean scar(s) or had my Caesarean scar(s) treated or I am taking care of
my Caesarean scar(s) / having my Caesarean scar(s) treated. no ☐   yes ☐, namely

_____

5.5)   It is easy for me to accept my Caesarean scar(s).   yes ☐   no ☐

5.6)   I find my Caesarean scar(s) ugly.   yes ☐   no ☐

5.7)   It is easy for me to touch my Caesarean scar(s).   yes ☐   no ☐

5.8)   My partner has a problem with my Caesarean (scar)s. no ☐   yes ☐, namely

_____

5.9)   My Caesarean scar(s) is/are (altogether) approx. _____ cm long.

5.10)   I would describe the shape of my Caesarean scar(s) as follows:

_____

5.11)   I would roughly sketch the appearance and position of my Caesarean scar(s) as follows on the picture:

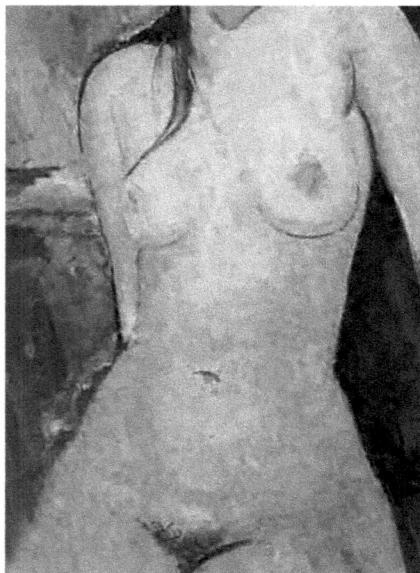

5.12)   What else comes to mind concerning my Caesarean
scar(s):

_____

_____

_____

_____

_____

_____

_____

_____

_____

_____

_____

6.1) I dealt with Caesareans intensively prior to my Caesarean.
no ☐   yes ☐, namely for this reason:

_____

_____

6.2) The Caesarean section was the ideal way of giving birth as far as I am concerned.
yes ☐   no ☐

6.3) I think that in future Caesarean section should generally replace vaginal birth.
yes ☐   no ☐

6.4) My Caesarean birth is seen as a fully-fledged birth / My Caesarean births are seen as fully-fledged births by my family, friends and acquaintances.
yes ☐   no ☐, this is expressed as follows:

_____

_____

6.5) Society gives me the feeling of having failed.
yes ☐   no ☐

6.6) In my opinion a Caesarean birth has negative effects on the child.
no ☐   yes ☐, namely the following:

_____

_____

6.7) I find that Caesarean section is trivialised and minimised by the media (newspaper, magazines, television, ...).   yes ☐   no ☐

6.8) I believe that the following reasons are responsible for the increase in Caesarean births:

_____

_____

6.9) My fundamental attitude on the topic "Caesarean" could be described as follows:

_____

_____

_____

_____

_____

_____

_____

_____

_____

_____

Questionnaire for obstetric experts:

Questions with a check box were to be marked with a cross, for questions to be answered freely an extra sheet of lined paper was available. Original format DIN A4.

Supplying personal data is optional and simply allows us to contact you in the case of a follow-up enquiry. All personal data will be made anonymous before publication.

1.) Personal data.

1.1) Surname / First name _____ 1.2) Title _____

1.3) Address _____

1.4) Phone number _____

1.5) E-mail address _____

2.) Statistical data.

2.1) Female ☐ Male ☐

2.2) Date of birth: _____._____.19_____

2.3) Occupation midwife ☐ gynaecologist ☐ physician ☐
other ☐: _____

2.4) I was delivered by Caesarean section myself. yes ☐ no ☐

2.5) My mother was delivered by Caesarean section. yes ☐ no ☐

2.6) I am a mother myself and have given birth to a total of _____ child(ren)
and had _____ Caesarean section(s).

3.) When I hear the word "Caesarean section" the following 5 words come to mind spontaneously:

3.1) 1. _____

3.2) 2. _____

3.3) 3. _____

3.4) 4. _____

3.5) 5. _____

4.) The Caesarean section from a medical point of view.

4.1)   A Caesarean section should definitely be performed for the following indications:

_____

_____

4.2)   A Caesarean section usually proceeds without complications.
yes ☐   no ☐, the following complications often occur:

_____

_____

4.3)   Nowadays the decision for a Caesarean section is mostly made by the following person(s):
(multiple answers possible)
physician ☐   midwife ☐   mother ☐   other ☐: _____

4.4)   The occurrence of real (natural) contractions before birth is important for the child and should
be awaited if possible.   yes ☐   no ☐

4.5)   Artificial/induced labour / contractions caused by drugs increase the chance of having to end
the birth with a Caesarean section.   yes ☐   no ☐

4.6)   If possible the Caesarean section should be performed under the following anaesthesia:
spinal anaesthesia ☐   epidural anaesthesia ☐
general anaesthesia ☐   other ☐: _____

5.) The Caesarean section and its consequences for mother and child.

5.1)   A Caesarean section is easy on mother and child and therefore better than a vaginal delivery.
yes ☐   no ☐

5.2)   In future Caesarean section should generally replace vaginal birth.   yes ☐   no ☐

5.3)   A Caesarean section has negative effects on the child.
no ☐   yes ☐, namely the following:

_____

_____

5.4)   A Caesarean section interferes with the mother-child bonding/relationship.
no ☐   yes ☐, namely for this reason:

_____

_____

5.5)   A previous Caesarean is often the indication for a repeat Caesarean section.   yes ☐   no ☐

5.6)   After two previous Caesareans a third Caesarean section is mandatory with a new pregnancy.
yes ☐   no ☐

5.7)   After three Caesarean sections the patient should have a tubal ligation.   yes ☐   no ☐

6.1)   The Caesarean section is a   birth ☐   surgery ☐

6.2)   I think that these days many Caesarean sections are performed without urgent medical indication.
        no ☐   yes ☐, namely for this reason:

        _____

        _____

6.3)   In my opinion an elective Caesarean requested by the woman should be performed even without
        medical indication.   yes ☐   no ☐

6.4)   I feel that Caesarean sections are more often performed during the day (7 a.m – 7 p.m) than
        outside of this time.   yes ☐   no ☐

6.5)   I think that women who have a private supplementary health insurance, deliver by Caesarean
        section more often.   yes ☐   no ☐

6.6)   Women with a higher educational level (A-levels, academic studies, ...) have an above average
        Cesarean rate.   yes ☐   no ☐

6.7)   I think that famous Caesarean mothers have a great influence on the rise in the rate of Caesareans.
                                                                         yes ☐   no ☐

6.8)   I find that Caesarean section is trivialised and minimised by the media (newspaper, magazines,
        television, ...).   yes ☐   no ☐

6.9)   My fundamental attitude on the topic "Caesarean" could be described as follows:

        _____

        _____

        _____

        _____

        _____

        _____

        _____

        _____

        _____

        _____

        _____

        _____

        _____

        _____

        _____

        _____

I have read this book.

I am a Caesarean mother too

My personal Caesarean questionnaire.

I have given birth to _____ child(ren), (_____ of them) by Caesarean section.

Occupation: _____

When I hear the word "Caesarean section" the following words come to mind spontaneously:

1. _____

2. _____

3. _____

4. _____

5. _____

The birth of my child(ren):

_____

_____

_____

_____

_____

_____

_____

_____

_____

_____

_____

The indication(s) for my section(s):

_____

_____

_____

_____

Was I afraid of pain during birth/of perineal trauma?

_____

Would I have preferred a vaginal delivery?

_____

Was the Caesarean the ideal way of giving birth for me?

_____

Did I experience the Caesarean section as traumatic?

_____

Does society give me the feeling of having failed?

_____

My opinion on the topic "Caesarean":

_____

_____

_____

_____

My Caesarean scar(s) is/are approx. _____ cm long.

Do I feel my Caesarean scar(s)? _____

Do I find my Caesarean scar(s) ugly? _____

Did I take care of it / treat it / have it treated? _____

Photograph

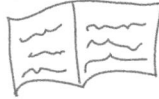

edition riedenburg

www.editionriedenburg.at

Buchreihen

Ich weiß jetzt wie! Reihe für Kinder bis ins Schulalter
SOWAS! – Kinder- und Jugend-Spezialsachbuchreihe
Verschiedene Alben für verwaiste Eltern und Geschwister

Einzeltitel

Alle meine Tage – Menstruationskalender
Alle meine Zähne – Zahnkalender für Kinder
Annikas andere Welt – Psychisch kranke Eltern
Ausgewickelt! So gelingt der Abschied von der Windel
Baby Lulu kann es schon! – Windelfreies Baby
Babymützen selbstgemacht! Ganz einfach ohne Nähen
Besonders wenn sie lacht – Lippen-Kiefer-Gaumenspalte
Bitterzucker – Nierentransplantation
Brüt es aus! Die freie Schwangerschaft
C-Section Moms – Caesarean mothers in words and photographs
Das doppelte Mäxchen – Zwillinge
Das große Storchenmalbuch mit Hebamme Maja
Der Kaiserschnitt hat kein Gesicht – Fotobuch
Der Wuschelfloh, der fliegt aufs Klo! – Spatz ohne Windel
Die Josefsgeschichte – Biblisches von Kindern für Kinder
Die Sonne sucht dich – Foto-Meditation Schwangerschaft
Drei Nummern zu groß – Kleinwuchs
Egal wie klein und zerbrechlich – Erinnerungsalbum
Ein Baby in unserer Mitte – Hausgeburt und Stillen
Finja kriegt das Fläschchen – Für Mamas, die nicht stillen
Frauenkastration – Fachwissen und Frauen-Erfahrungen
Ich war ein Wolfskind aus Königsberg – DDR und BRD
In einer Stadt vor unserer Zeit – Regensburg-Reiseführer
Jutta juckt's nicht mehr – Hilfe bei Neurodermitis
Konrad, der Konfliktlöser – Clever streiten und versöhnen
Lass es raus! Die freie Geburt
Leg dich nieder! Das freie Wochenbett
Lilly ist ein Sternenkind – Verwaiste Geschwister
Lorenz wehrt sich – Sexueller Missbrauch

Luxus Privatgeburt – Hausgeburten in Wort und Bild
Machen wie die Großen – Rund ums Klogehen
Maharishi Good Bye – Tiefenmeditation und die Folgen
Mama und der Kaiserschnitt – Kaiserschnitt
Mamas Bauch wird kugelrund – Aufklärung für Kinder
Manchmal verlässt uns ein Kind – Erinnerungsalbum
Mein Sternenkind – Verwaiste Eltern
Meine Folgeschwangerschaft – Schwanger nach Verlust
Meine Wunschgeburt – Gebären nach Kaiserschnitt
Mit Liebe berühren – Erinnerungsalbum
Mord in der Oper – Bellinis letzter Vorhang
Nasses Bett? – Nächtliches Einnässen
Nino und die Blumenwiese – Nächtliches Einnässen, Bilderbuch
Oma braucht uns – Pflegebedürftige Angehörige
Oma war die Beste! – Trauerfall in der Familie
Papa in den Wolken-Bergen – Verlust eines nahen Angehörigen
Pauline purzelt wieder – Übergewichtige Kinder
Regelschmerz ade! Die freie Menstruation
So klein, und doch so stark! – Extreme Frühgeburt
So leben wir mit Endometriose – Hilfe für betroffene Frauen
Soloschläfer – Erholsamer Mutter-Kind-Schlaf ohne Mann
Still die Badewanne voll! Das freie Säugen
Stille Brüste – Das Fotobuch für die Stillzeit und danach
Tragekinder – Das Kindertragen Kindern erklärt
Und der Klapperstorch kommt doch! – Kinderwunsch
Und wenn du dich getröstet hast – Erinnerungsalbum
Unser Baby kommt zu Hause! – Hausgeburt
Unser Klapperstorch kugelt rum! – Schwangerschaft
Unsere kleine Schwester Nina – Babys erstes Jahr
Volle Hose – Einkoten bei Kindern